THE FEELING OVERRIDES NUTRITION

By DanM@CowsEatGrass

Copyright 2022, by DanM@CowsEatGrass. All rights reserved. This copyright protects author-publisher DanM@CowsEatGrass's right to future publication of his work in any manner, in all media — utilising technology now known or devised — throughout the world in perpetuity. Everything described in this publication is for information purposes only.

The author-publisher, DanM@CowsEatGrass, is not a medical doctor and does not directly or indirectly present or recommend any part of this publication's data as a diagnosis or prescription for any medical, psychological, or other ailments of any reader. Suppose anyone uses this information without the advice of their professional health adviser. In that case, they are prescribing for themselves, and the author-publisher assumes no responsibility or liability. Persons using this data do so at their own risk and must take personal responsibility for what they don't know and for what they do know.

The content of this book is not a substitute for advice from a healthcare professional. And it would be best if you did not disregard medical advice. Nor should you delay seeking it due to opinions, recommendations or any other information you have read in this book.

The opinions expressed within this book are the opinions of the author. To the extent permitted by law, the author assumes no liability or responsibility for damage or injury to persons or property arising from any use of information, ideas, or opinions found within this book.

Mind is the forerunner of all states. Mind is chief; mind-made are they.

Dhammapada Verse 1-20 (The Twins)

What follows was inspired by the teachings of the Buddha and is dedicated to Venerable Bhante Vimalaramsi who has shown so many what the Buddha really taught about relief from suffering, that science is still catching up with.

Table Of Contents

Preface

Introduction

Part One Recognising The Feeling

Chapter 1 / Mind Body Mind Body

Chapter 2 / Your Mind On A Diet

Chapter 3 / It's Just A Feeling

Chapter 4 / The Second Layer

Chapter 5 / Irritable Mind Syndrome

Chapter 6 / The Tides Of Conceiving

Chapter 7 / What Does This Feeling Mean?

Chapter 8 / You Can't Think Away A Feeling

Chapter 9 / Three "Noble" Metabolic Truths

Part Two Dealing With The Feeling

Chapter 10 / All Pain Is Not Suffering

Chapter 11 / Fix Your Energy Fix Your Thyroid

Chapter 12 / Imperfect Perfect Health

Chapter 13 / Replacing Pathways To Stress

Chapter 14 / Feed Metabolism Not Stress

Chapter 15 / PTSDissipation

Chapter 16 / Look, Let Go, Digest

Chapter 17 / Everybody Needs Attention

Chapter 18 / Default To Happiness

Chapter 19 / Relaxing Metabolic Craving

Chapter 20 / The Buddha's Metabolism

Chapter 21 / Cool Heat

Chapter 22 / Making Your System Nervous

Chapter 23 / What Me Worry About

Chapter 24 / Stress MetHabitolism

Chapter 25 / "80% Perfect"

Chapter 26 / Symptoms Not Suffering

Chapter 27 / Fear Of Fear

Chapter 28 / The Future Is Now

Chapter 29 / Habitual Pathways

Chapter 30 / Smiling Lowers Serotonin

Chapter 31 / Serious Anxiety And Depression

Chapter 32 / Reverse Superstition

Chapter 33 / Pain Is Impermanent

Chapter 34 / Catch a Bad Mood

Chapter 35 / Which Meditation?

Preface

THE TITLE OF the book came to me one afternoon early in 2021 while contemplating the link between stress and metabolism and why diet and lifestyle changes seem to work so much better for some than others. For a long time, I thought the reason was that they just needed to get their diet and lifestyle right. But my own experiences with using such methods to improve metabolism taught me that there must be more to it than that.

I started learning about nutrition a few decades ago when training in martial arts. I suffered from bouts of anxiety and depression for as long as I can remember, and my interest in martial arts came from a desire to solve these issues. However, the more I trained, the more I realised it wouldn't be easy. I began to suffer from digestion problems and several other things.

In my early 40s, it became clear that martial arts training and competition greatly strained my body and mind. I was barely coping physically and mentally, even though I felt I had found many ways to improve my health significantly through dietary changes. I needed to find a better solution, and found it in yoga.

But again, the stress of life continued to take its toll, and I started to think there was no way to get the result I wanted. It felt as though no matter what I did to improve my health and happiness, something in me always got in my way. So this book came from my search to find what that thing is. It turns out that it was something very subtle and yet highly significant.

Thank you to Alexandra for all her help with the editing process, for listening to my ideas, and for letting me have my tent in her living room.

For more of my work, go to www.CowsEatGrass.org

Introduction

It's not uncommon to hear it said that happiness depends on good health and that poor health causes suffering. It's difficult to dispute that a well-functioning system provides advantages. Still, I'm going to let you in on a little secret. It isn't truly a secret, but it needs to get discussed more because it's easy to forget, especially when it needs remembering most.

What it is is that many people who aren't lucky enough to have good health still manage to live meaningful, joyful and happiness-filled lives. So it is worth saying, perhaps twice, and remembering.

The fact is, nowhere is it stated that a life without health issues is guaranteed. Unfortunately, not all physiological problems can be avoided or fixed. Whether a person knows nothing about nutrition, or even if they have a PhD in pro-metabolic eating, you can rely on one thing. At some point in life, everybody will face health problems.

Still, it's understandable why having good health is considered essential. Poor health is painful, limiting, inconvenient and fear-inducing, as well as many other challenging and unpleasant things. And because poor health doesn't feel good, it also interferes with happiness. And then unhappiness can interfere with metabolism, making poor health worse.

This book is about health and healing but isn't a guidebook for achieving perfect metabolism. Instead, it's a book about why improving nutrition or lifestyle can fail to work as well as hoped regarding health and happiness. In fact, for some, it's counter-productive, and probably not for the reasons you think.

One important reason is that the desire to attain good health can become a mission to achieve perfect health. But unfortunately, this can end up becoming a hindrance to health and happiness. That's in no small part because there isn't such a thing as "perfect health" to be achieved. But I'll get into that further down the track.

Yes, health is essential. Therefore, learning how to improve metabolism with nutrition or lifestyle changes is a worthwhile passtime. And I have passed much time away on these endeavours.

This book is still a book about healing metabolic function. But more accurately, it's a book about *The Feeling*, how people interact with it, and how it relates to metabolism, health, and happiness.

What is *The Feeling,* I hear you ask? You might have to hold on because I've gotten ahead of myself. All will get revealed in good time.

But while we're on metabolic health, let me ask you this. Do you wonder why some do well under suboptimal conditions, and others tweak their diet or lifestyle program into something out of a NASA handbook, still feeling average? If you guessed that I'm going to suggest this has something to do with metabolism, you're on the right track.

You might already know (if you've read anything I've written) that metabolism impacts health and happiness, and diet and lifestyle influence metabolic conditions. And people are gifted with various metabolic performance or resilience levels, influencing their system's sensitivity to foods and stressful activities and environments.

Excess stress exposure (including environmental toxins like estrogenic chemicals and radiation) interferes with metabolism, impacting digestion and changing how you handle stress. Of course, there's a lot you can tweak with all this to improve health and happiness, and there's usually more than one thing that comes into play regarding how a person feels, physically and mentally.

But what happens if you don't get the results you want? What if you've tried everything and are still unhappy? What if you want to feel better and be happier? Then what? That's a big part of this book and has everything to do with *The Feeling*.

Part One Recognising The Feeling

Chapter 1 / Mind Body Mind Body

How do you feel? It's a question people get asked all the time. But the question is, is it the right question? Has anybody asked you lately *how you feel about how you feel*? No, I didn't think so. But you'll see, this question is a far more critical question, and it's what this book will explore. That's right, *how you feel about how you feel*. And how this has a significant influence on how you feel.

I know it sounds obvious or even silly, but I promise you there's more to it than meets the eye. *How you feel about how you feel* impacts how you feel and does so in a way that how you feel doesn't. And no, saying it like that won't automatically clear it up. But, don't worry, we'll get there eventually, and you'll be happy when we do.

You might already have realised that *how you feel about how you feel* has something to do with the mind-body. Or, in other words, the intertwined nature of mind and body. The mind-body is not a discovery. It's common knowledge that (to the extent that mind and body are separate entities) the mind impacts the body, and the body impacts the mind. It's hard to argue with that. Most people know it to be true in one way or another. But knowing it's true doesn't automatically fix all issues.

Still, it's an excellent place to start because knowing about the mind-body can lead to powerful insights regarding metabolism and health. One such understanding is that improvements in the mind or the body equate to improvements in metabolism. Another insight is that fixing one metabolic issue helps fix other metabolic problems because that's how the mind-body and metabolism work.

You will find that most early insights regarding how this system functions focus on tweaking diet and lifestyle to improve the quality of communication between mind and body. And knowing how to enhance mind-body communication will improve how you feel, but *how you feel about how you feel* is another story, as you will find out.

But the more you know how the mind and body are interrelated, the better you understand metabolism, opening up a new way of looking at what you consume and do daily. When you learn how to use diet and lifestyle to improve metabolism, mysteries regarding what causes seemingly unrelated health/happiness problems that perplexed you for a long time unravel.

After years of experimenting with nutrition, I stumbled on the work of Dr Ray Peat. It helped me improve many of my "separate, unrelated, puzzling, inexplicable, no reason, psychosomatic" issues. Chronic digestive distress, anxiety, depression, insomnia, lack of energy, skin inflammation, infections and other problems that came and went for seemingly no common reason all improved dramatically after making changes based on a pro-metabolic mind-body approach. It was a pretty big deal.

But before you get this lucky, you can spend a decade restricting sugar, avoiding salt and saturated fats, and assaulting your intestines with under-cooked vegetable matter, tofu, chickpeas, plus loads of seeds, nuts and weeds. Not to mention the "heart healthy" PUFAs, which include the wondrous "anti-inflammatory Omega-3s".

And you won't just be wading through suboptimal diet information. Instead, you'll often get vague platitudes regarding lifestyle/mindset changes for improving metabolism or mind-body communication.

Indeed, changing your outlook and behaviours can enormously impact overall happiness and metabolic function. But, sadly, new age mantras like "see each setback as an opportunity" or "connect to the moment and allow your subconscious to create inner safety" give false hope and worse.

And although potentially beneficial, advice to exercise or to go outside and interact with nature also creates new variables (and new questions) and results that vary from person to person. And state-of-the-art neurophysiology drills, authentic yoga instruction, breathing techniques and meditation or relaxation methods can also improve mind-body performance. Again, results vary.

But even when these approaches promote the healing of metabolism, they only improve how you feel up to a point. Because they fail to deal with *how you feel about how you feel*, and you need to deal with it.

It's easy to think how you feel is just one big "the way you feel". But it isn't like that. It gets made up of parts. Some parts make up how you feel, and some parts make up *how you feel about how you feel*, and *how you feel about how you feel* can change how you feel in a big way.

Chapter 2 / Your Mind On A Diet

If you know me, you'll know I'm not a great believer in diets per se. But something must also get said about putting your mind on a diet. It has to do with nutrients, but mostly it has to do with nutriments. Some years ago, as a student and practitioner of yoga, I came across the Hatha Yoga Pradipika, a classic fifteenth-century Sanskrit manual on haṭha yoga.

In the years leading up to that, I immersed myself in the writings of Dr Ray Peat. Doing so resulted in drastic changes to my eating habits and my understanding of the impact of nutrition and lifestyle on metabolic performance. So I was surprised to read in the Hatha Yoga Pradipika that the diet for a yogi, the sattvic way of eating (mitāhārah), includes easy-to-digest sweet foods and dairy products, similar to what I was already doing.

> *Abstemious feeding is that in which 3⁄4 of hunger is satisfied with food, well cooked with ghee and sweets, and eaten with the offering of it to Śiva.*
>
> *Wheat, rice, barley, shâstik (a kind of rice), good corns, milk, ghee, sugar, butter, sugarcandy, honey, dried ginger, Parwal (a vegetable) the five vegetables, moong, pure water; these are very beneficial to those who practise Yoga* (Hatha Yoga Pradipika).

My way of eating at the time (and still to this day), inspired by my interpretation of the writings of Dr Peat, was designed to achieve stress reduction and improved metabolic function. It primarily consisted of milk, cheese, orange juice, sugar, and other ingredients, serving me well. This pro-metabolic way significantly reduced symptoms I had suffered from on and off for a few decades, relating to digestion and mood.

The combination of a pro-metabolic dietary approach and yoga practice was taking on a synergistic quality, allowing me to do things that would previously have seemed unthinkable. Finally, I realised yoga, combined with a yogic way of eating, is far more powerful and effective. It also became apparent that a pro-metabolic approach aligned with the principles of biology and metabolism and with ancient yogic teachings.

I witnessed first-hand how a sattvic way of eating assists in promoting a sattvic state of mind and how a sattvic state of mind then promotes metabolic equilibrium.

> *Of all the restrictive rules, that relating to the taking of sattvic food in moderate quantities is the best; by observing this rule, the sattvic quality of mind will increase, and that will be helpful to Self-inquiry (*Who Am I? The Teachings of Bhagavan Sri Ramana Maharshi).

What is a sattvic state of mind? It is a calm, relaxed, wholesome, self-aware mind. My mind moved in a sattvic direction, and my views on how metabolic improvement influences the state of mind also shifted. A sattvic mind is in equilibrium, a mind in the middle.

When the body is in equilibrium, the mind also moves toward equilibrium. As a result, the mind-body becomes more stable.

My experience (from a reasonably well-controlled self-experiment) showed me that diet and lifestyle changes reduce stress and improve happiness.

Fruit, dairy and sugar are particularly effective because they promote metabolism and equilibrium. They improve energy production and digestion, protecting against stress and inflammation. I learned that improved metabolism means equilibrium.

But that wasn't all I learned. I began to notice how an equanimous mind state calms metabolism. I saw improved digestive performance and greater resilience to mental and emotional stress. I discovered that a sattvic state of mind is less fazed by stress. A mind less fazed by stress is also a body less fazed by stress. So it builds a metabolism that can better meet stress with thyroid energy.

A system in equilibrium is relaxed and can provide more energy for digestion. Although today it's considered extreme to have a diet centred around dairy, fruit and sugar, an approach promoting metabolism is a dietary middle way. The sattvic way of eating is a nutritional precursor for a more neutral, even state of mind, less fazed by the arising of a good or a bad feeling. It promotes balance mentally and physically. I soon learned, however, that even when you dial in diet and lifestyle, life continues to provide stress, things still go wrong in the body, and the mind feeds on more than just food.

What does the mind feed on? It is an important question. Even if the body gets optimal nutrition, the mind is constantly consuming, and what the mind consumes affects both the mind and the body. It is nutriments that the mind feeds on, and this includes more than just nutrition. It includes everything the mind feeds on. That means anything the mind comes into contact with, like sounds, smells, sights, thoughts, emotions and sensations. What you eat and do with your body impacts your state of mind, but that's far from the end of the story. It's closer to the beginning.

If your mind is calm, that calms metabolic function. It will calm digestion, for example, and reduce exposure to stress substances like serotonin and nitric oxide, which, in excess, interfere with metabolic function and state of mind. Eating stress-lowering metabolism-promoting foods is one way to improve the ability to assimilate food in the intestines, which helps calm the mind. Relaxation techniques and nervous system recalibration techniques are other powerful ways.

But the diet your mind is on, made up of everything the mind interacts with, has the power to create conditions that limit the effectiveness of a pro-metabolic diet and lifestyle. What your mind feeds on directly impacts how you feel, so it's natural to want to try to control what your mind consumes. But is it always possible?

Even if you move to the top of a mountain, live in a cave, or become a monk or a nun, your mind will come with you. And your mind will continue to find things to feed on because that's what minds do. So you can be in the most peaceful place; the tiniest thing can set your mind off. Then, before you know it, you're lost in thought. And then, before you know it, you're irritated, angry, lonely, in pain, anxious, depressed, or even in a state of panic.

And all this impacts metabolism. So if the mind is stressed, the body will be stressed, and the next thing you know, the mind is feeding on that, and a vicious circle can get set in motion. So when the mind is stressed, that immediately interferes with digestion having a powerful impact on metabolism and then on the mind again.

The reverse is also true. A calm wholesome state of mind improves digestion, intestinal barrier, and liver function.

The improved liver function reduces exposure to bacterial endotoxin, serotonin, estrogen, nitric oxide, and many other metabolism-interfering substances. Less interference with metabolism leads to protection from depression and other issues affecting the mind. It can often mean less suffering and more happiness.

All this is great to know about because it can improve how you feel, but often less than hoped for. Because there's another part of the diet your mind is on that is not seen, that is, the part to do with *how you feel about how you feel*. And that part needs to be addressed. *How you feel about how you feel* is made up of processes in the mind-body. They interact with the diet your mind is on. But the interactions that determine how your mind's diet impacts *how you feel about how you feel* are easily missed.

Chapter 3 / It's Just A Feeling

When a feeling arises in the mind-body, that's all it is, a feeling. But that's rarely the end of it. Instead, what happens after a feeling changes everything, for better or worse. Well, more often for worse. So what exactly happens?

Whether a feeling is bad or whether it's good doesn't matter. The answer is the same. Lots of things happen. Lots of rapidly moving things, and most people don't notice them, not at least until after you tell them to watch out for them.

I like to refer to them as layers because, looking more carefully, you'll see that layers get added to a feeling turning it into *The Feeling*. Of course, even smaller parts make up these layers, but that's a story for another time. The critical question is, do you need to look for anything in particular?

The answer is yes; you need to look out for *The Feeling*. *The Feeling* can be any feeling you notice in the mind-body because even after it becomes *The Feeling,* it's still just a feeling. So to be clear, you need to look out for a feeling, and it doesn't matter what type of feeling. Just something that you feel. There's nothing special about it. Even when a feeling arises (before it becomes *The Feeling*), that's not the beginning. Instead, it's connected to other layers that took place before. But I digress. What's important is that the moment you notice a feeling is when you need to because that's when you did. So whether it's a feeling or *The Feeling* is not what matters. It's what you do with it that makes or breaks you.

So it can be any feeling you notice. It can be pain, nausea, discomfort, anxiety, weakness, dizziness, pressure, overheating, fear, sadness, or anything else you can feel (including a good feeling). As I said, it doesn't matter.

A feeling can arise from metabolic fluctuations, an experience, the environment, or many other reasons. Why it appeared is not the issue either. What makes a feeling become *The Feeling* has nothing to do with the feeling it is. Any feeling can become *The Feeling*. The difference between the two is a different kind of difference.

A pro-metabolic approach says that what makes a feeling arise determines what kind of feeling it is, which is responsible for how it makes you feel. So figure out what made it occur, deal with that, and then do more of what causes a better feeling. Hopefully, eventually, you will feel how you want to feel. Every feeling indeed gets created out of causes and conditions. These causes and conditions include the state of your metabolism, stress exposure levels, diet, lifestyle and other choices, and many things outside your control. Therefore, a feeling can feel good, and a feeling can feel bad.

And it's true knowing what causes a feeling to arise can help improve how you feel. That's what a pro-metabolic diet and lifestyle are about. But we'll be exploring what happens after a feeling arises that transforms it from being a feeling into the problem known as *The Feeling*. So what makes a feeling arise in the first place is not the issue.

No matter what makes a feeling arise or what kind of feeling it is, it can become *The Feeling* or remain just a feeling. And *The Feeling* still is just a feeling, even though it has changed into something very different. That might not sound very clear, but it will become clear. So let's move on.

When a feeling arises, it can become *The Feeling* very rapidly. So rapidly that you miss it. But whether you see it happening or not, layers are added to it to make this happen. Suppose you don't know about the added layers when you notice a feeling. In that case, all you'll see is one immense feeling, coming and going, growing or shrinking. And you'll have explanations for why this is happening. Then if somebody asks you how you feel, your answer won't just be about how you feel. It'll include *how you feel about how you feel*, at no extra charge. That's "the full catastrophe". *The Feeling* is a full catastrophe feeling, and a full catastrophe feeling is much more challenging. It causes more unhappiness (and health issues) than just a feeling. Just this difference can create a world of suffering.

The Feeling can be overwhelming and feel like it has a life of its own. It's still just a feeling, but now you feel worse, and there are probably more bad feelings on their way. So what to do? Let's say you notice a feeling arising, and it's a feeling you don't like. The first thing you need to know is that it's here. You didn't ask for it to be here, but it's here, and that's a fact. So no matter what you think of it or why you think it's here, it's here.

Maybe overeating gave you a stomach ache, or you got invited out and feel anxious about going, or perhaps you have a pain in the body and are worried about it. A feeling has arisen, and that's reality. Whether or not you want it to be here, you can't know how long it will stay. You're aware of it, and that's all there is to it.

Now don't be disheartened. It is good news. You're on the way to understanding the difference between a feeling and *The Feeling*. And this is where the power lies. The power doesn't come from fixing a feeling or even from fixing *The Feeling*. So feel free to do that. Call a doctor, change your diet, do a headstand, jump in cold water or whatever else you like. That's up to you, and there's nothing wrong with that. But even if those things help, knowing what happens once a feeling has arisen to turn it into *The Feeling* has untapped power. And even if it's already *The Feeling,* the power works.

So what happens after a feeling arises that has the power to harm or help? Let me tell you. When a feeling arises, you perceive something about it. Then, either you don't like it and want it to go, or you like it and want it to stay. That's it. That's the beginning of turning a feeling into *The Feeling*. It doesn't sound like much, but it's very much.

Not knowing this causes a world of suffering. But knowing just this one thing can take you from suffering to freedom. Freedom doesn't mean a bad feeling won't arise anymore. On the contrary, there will still be pain (and pleasure), but something big happens. You'll be happier, and even though there will be metabolic issues, this freedom can improve metabolism as a byproduct.

But if you don't know about this, a feeling will likely become *The Feeling*, and all you'll see is one big problem that needs to be dealt with to be healthy and happy again.

Yes, an arising feeling can be a sign of suboptimal metabolism. And yes, the worse a feeling feels, the more it stresses metabolism. But this isn't just about a bad feeling. A pleasant feeling feels good. You like it, and you want it to stay. You want more. You don't want less. In that way, it is like a bad feeling, only inverted. Both scenarios are a recipe for less happiness and more dissatisfaction.

It's what the world's most famous meditation teacher, Gotama Buddha, called *craving*. A meditation guide of mine, Venerable Bhante Vimalaramsi, calls it the "I like it, I don't like it mind".

> *Now what's the definition of craving? It's the mind that says 'I like it' or 'I don't like it'. OK, the 'I like it, I don't like it mind' is craving. A painful feeling arises and that craving feeling is right there saying I don't like it. I don't want it to be there. I want it to stop. I don't like this pain. I don't like this suffering.* (Ven. Bhante Vimalaramsi)

Liking or disliking a feeling happens as soon as a feeling arises, and it causes suffering. It limits happiness and impacts metabolism. According to the Buddha, *craving* is responsible for endless suffering, and it's a key to ending suffering.

On the one hand, a feeling tells you something about metabolism, which can be helpful up to a point. But on the other hand, a feeling is just a feeling, and whether you understand why it's there or not, it's there whether or not you like it. Even when you think you know why it's there, you don't necessarily understand why, so how you fix it can backfire. Still, if a feeling has arisen, it has arisen, and if it has gone away, it has gone away.

You can respond to a feeling arising in two ways. You can let it be a feeling or create *The Feeling*. How you feel is just a feeling. *How you feel about how you feel* turns it into *The Feeling*. *The Feeling* is more than just a feeling; it is "your feeling". It's personal now, and that's what makes all the difference. And it's like the difference between day and night or a nightmare.

Chapter 4 / The Second Layer

"I don't like this feeling. I want it to go". Alternatively, "I like this feeling. I want it to stay". Once the mind-body knows it doesn't like a feeling, or once it knows it likes a feeling, this is the second layer. And the second layer can create an endless amount of suffering.

Regardless, it's natural to think that when a feeling arises, it's what is responsible for how you feel. And it's natural to focus on that. But it isn't to blame. It's just a feeling, after all. And the jump from just a feeling to "I don't like it" (or "I like it") happens so rapidly that it's barely noticeable. Almost nobody notices it.

So what starts as just a feeling gets a layer added to it, making it feel different. What is this layer made of? This layer gets made up of dissatisfaction with a feeling that comes with tension or a contraction in the mind-body. The combination is called *craving*.

Because you aren't aware it's happening, you get taken away, and all that seems to exist is a more substantial feeling. So the added layer escapes detection. It increases the intensity of a feeling. And that has a real impact on metabolism. So the added stress is real, and the effect on happiness is too.

The *craving* feeds the expansion of a feeling. The combination of tension and dissatisfaction interferes with the ability to see a feeling for what it is. It's just a feeling, but it feels like more. It feels like "your feeling"; or like you are what you feel. But it is only a feeling. It is part of you, but you are more than that. More on that later. For now, no matter how many layers get added, no matter how personal and powerful it gets, it's never not just a feeling. But it expands rapidly, and all it takes is the addition of just that one layer of *how you feel about how you feel*. Do ya feel me?

And just like how you can transform a feeling into *The Feeling*, you can go back to a feeling being just a feeling, and that's the beginning of seeing things how they are. The earlier you see the transformation, the more suffering and unhappiness can be averted. Sorry to inform you that it rarely gets seen early.

The more how you feel gets influenced by *how you feel about how you feel*, the bigger *The Feeling* gets and the harder it is to deal with it. And the more it affects metabolism. There are physiological explanations for a feeling, but *how you feel about how you feel* can't be measured in a lab. For example, c*raving* does not show up on a blood test.

These layers exist outside mainstream biology and have suffering and unhappiness built into them. But these processes are not separate from biology. So the pain, discomfort, nausea, anxiety, sadness, anger, or anything else coming off an expanding feeling can make you sicker than you were.

Dissatisfaction with a feeling is not all bad. There's a good reason not to keep your hand on the flame, swallow more poison, or get heatstroke. And there's good reason to want sugar, although most would disagree. Instinctive protection reactions help you make decisions for the sake of personal safety. But a worsening feeling is not necessarily protecting you from danger. Often the size and intensity of a feeling increase due to factors unrelated to harm avoidance; this causes harm.

It's just one little layer, but it opens you up to a world of unhappiness and metabolic interference. But, on the flip side, knowing about it can open you up to a great opportunity. The good news is that taking advantage of this opportunity isn't complicated; it's simple. You only have to know what to watch out for and practice watching. It is exciting news. Only don't get too excited. Before I tell you how simple it is to practice, there's some more you need to know.

Chapter 5 / Irritable Mind Syndrome

There's a direct link between the mind and metabolism, especially with the digestive system. So whenever the mind is tense, digestion will likely not be optimal. And when digestion isn't optimal, many things feel worse, including the state of mind. And this can quickly become a vicious circle.

How you feel about how you feel is dissatisfaction added to a feeling plus the tension that comes with that, referred to by the Buddha as *craving*. The Buddha said *craving* is what's at the heart of unnecessary suffering. And it turns out that's a large percentage of suffering. But if that's not bad enough, something worse happens, directly on top of *craving*—the next layer.

The next layer is a reaction to *craving*. It's known in Buddhism as *clinging*, and it causes what I call Irritable Mind Syndrome. If you guessed this has to do with thinking, you guessed right. But not thoughts per se. Thoughts are a necessary and regular part of life. It has to do with repetitive or circular thinking that surrounds *craving*. If you think *how you feel about how you feel* makes a difference to how you feel, wait till you see what repetitive circular thinking does.

Let's say a feeling arises that you dislike and want to go. The dissatisfaction plus tension that comes with it is *craving*. The mind immediately reacts to *craving* with the next layer, thinking about why you don't like a feeling. It happens very quickly. The mind starts telling a story about why it's a bad feeling and how it means something is wrong. It can also be about how if you don't get rid of this feeling, you'll never get better, and things will worsen.

The details aren't the important thing. What matters is it's a feeling you don't like, it has tension going with it, and then the thoughts get added onto it. So now you're hyper-fixated on your beliefs about a feeling, which expands *The Feeling*. It started as just a feeling, and now it feels much worse, and because you aren't aware of this process, all you think's happening is that things are going downhill. Where that ends up going depends significantly on how far the story goes. And to think this all began with just a dissatisfactory feeling. Powerful stuff.

The problem has nothing to do with the thinking being a bad thing. On the contrary, thinking is useful, necessary and probably unavoidable. Trying to stop thinking can take you down a perilous path.

The problem now is still the same as earlier. You're unaware that how you feel turned into *The Feeling* because of *how you feel about how you feel*. And then *The Feeling* expands even more because of *what you think about how you feel*. It's still "just a feeling", but you've made it personal. It's that simple. So that's the next step, but it's the same fundamental problem. Only now, it makes you feel even worse.

The order things happen can vary. It can start with an irritated digestive system or mind. How you approach the situation doesn't have to change. Whether a sensation arises first or a thought doesn't matter; it's all mind anyway. If you tense up immediately and don't want it to be there (or don't want it to go away), you'll be thinking about why, and before you know it, you'll feel worse. Now that your thoughts are irritated, chances are your intestines are too.

And what happens next? You don't like how you feel; you get even tenser and start thinking more about the worsening situation. You're just trying to make yourself feel better, but because you aren't aware of how the process works, you make yourself feel worse.

> *When that feeling arises, you'll notice that the first thing is that your mind begins to think about it or tell a story why it's there. Why you like it? Why you don't like it? Why you want it to be different than it is? Why you want it to stop and go away? All of the thoughts about the feeling makes the feeling bigger and more intense.*
> (Venerable Bhante Vimalaramsi).

Thoughts aren't the problem here. But using thinking to make a feeling feel better can be a problem. It's an avoidance technique, and it almost always backfires. The thinking tricks you into thinking you're fixing a feeling, and your attention gets diverted away from it, making it feel like it's working. But this feeds a feeling and makes it bigger and stronger. It also hides a bigger truth, but more on that later.

It's no secret that repetitive thinking can increase stress and that excessive stress irritates the mind, metabolism, and digestion. Stress moves blood flow away from digestion into peripheral tissue and impedes intestinal barrier function. Stress also causes interference with the use of sugar for energy production and releases free fatty acids into circulation. It is all part of a metabolic avoidance strategy.

The substances that rise due to intestinal irritation (such as bacterial endotoxin, serotonin, nitric oxide and lactic acid) suppress metabolism, diverting from unmet stress. But suppression of metabolism and excessive exposure to stress substances can work like dysfunctional thinking because it can cause more problems than it solves, especially in the long run.

Irritable Mind Syndrome is a product of repetitive thinking that promotes systemic stress. In addition, it causes further suppression of energy metabolism, promoting increased exposure to the type of sensation often connected with depression or anxiety. I'm sure you can guess where this leads.

It leads to more personalisation, dissatisfaction and tension, followed by more thinking and then expansion of *The Feeling*. So now there's more suffering and more unhappiness. The point here is not to disregard pain in the gut or every thought about what action to take. There's a time to act (and think), but the expansion of *The Feeling* doesn't help and is avoidable. That is if you know how to avoid it.

For starters, what's required is an awareness of how and why the expansion is happening and when it's happening. Once you start the ball rolling, the rest will come naturally. Even so, I'm going to tell you the rest.

Chapter 6 / The Tides Of Conceiving

As you probably already know, a big part of what determines whether or not a person gets sick is their behaviour on a day-to-day basis. Not that sickness and health are under your control. Still, there are ways to improve or worsen how metabolism, the immune system, and the nervous system function, and these ways increase or decrease protection from disease.

Even when somebody eats the "right foods", avoids environmental toxins, or does the best exercises, illness can still happen. It's a fact of life, and there's no avoiding the realities of life.

But what is illness? The word has much power, sometimes even more power than meaning. It can mean many different things, and what you think it means changes how much power it has and how you feel. How bad you feel impacts metabolism. If nobody can tell you what your illness is, all you can do is describe how you feel.

So you say something changed in the mind-body, and whatever changed has led to a feeling that does not feel good. It's a feeling that you don't want to be there. The bigger or more unpleasant it is, the worse you will describe the illness.

Don't get me wrong. I'm not saying illness isn't a natural phenomenon. Being ill is very unpleasant. It can be uncomfortable, painful, limiting, exhausting, and other complex and challenging things. Nobody likes being sick.

To sum it up, the worst thing about illness is how it changes how you feel. But it doesn't only change that. It also changes *how you feel about how you feel*. And then it changes *what you think about how you feel*, releasing "the tides of conceiving". And the tides of conceiving will sweep over you if you don't know what's happening.

> '*The tides of conceiving do not sweep over one who stands upon these foundations, and when the tides of conceiving no longer sweep over him he is called a sage at peace.' So it was said. And with reference to what was this said? Bhikkhu, 'I am' is a conceiving; 'I am this' is a conceiving; 'I shall be' is a conceiving; 'I shall not be' is a conceiving; 'I shall be possessed of form' is a conceiving; 'I shall be formless' is a conceiving; 'I shall be percipient' is a conceiving; 'I shall be non-percipient' is a conceiving; 'I shall be neither-percipient-nor-non-percipient' is a conceiving. Conceiving is a disease, conceiving is a tumor, conceiving is a dart. By overcoming all conceivings, bhikkhu, one is called a sage at peace.*
> (Dhātuvibhaṅgasutta, Majjhima Nikāya).

So a feeling arises, and let's say, for the sake of argument, you don't like it, and you want it gone. The mind then starts running through reasons why you don't like it, why you need to make it go away, and what will happen if it doesn't. It's the third layer, known in Buddhism as *clinging*, and comes straight after *craving*. The mind is trying to gain control with thinking, but it's thinking taking control. So thoughts start to make up a more prominent component of what's causing dissatisfaction, plus the discontent is growing.

First, how you feel expands due to *how you feel about how you feel*, and then *what you think about how you feel* moves into the first place. And this makes you feel much worse because *The Feeling* is getting stronger. And sadly, there are still more layers to come. And all this happens so quickly that most people don't realise it's happening.

Even after you know about the layers, this process happens so fast that you'll continue to get involved without even realising you're getting involved. A feeling will arise, and you're dissatisfied without being aware. There's tension, and then you're thinking about it, and things are escalating. Who can say how much?

Your conditioning is to react to a feeling a certain way. The mind wants to control how you feel and thinks it can do that by thinking, even though the evidence shows otherwise. A feeling arises, but you don't make it occur. Then thoughts arise, and you don't make them happen either. So what makes you think you can control them?

There's nothing inherently wrong with a feeling or a thought. On the contrary, a feeling or a thought can sometimes be instrumental. The problem starts when you make a feeling or thought into your feeling or thought. Then, it's no longer just a feeling or thought. It's personal. It becomes your identity. It's the story of you, but it isn't entirely true. It's *The Feeling*.

Liking or disliking is personal, and then building a story on top of that also is, but the truth is impersonal. So personalising or identifying with a feeling is what makes it a problem. Personalising causes the tides of conceiving to sweep over you. "I don't like how it feels. My pain is getting worse. I am sick. I shall get sicker. I am not getting better." When the tides sweep over you, you can drown in them.

Even though a feeling or a thought isn't personal, if you treat it like it is and try to control it, the mind-body responds to it like it is, amplifying its power. When you feel run down, have a runny nose or a headache, or feel tired, weak or overheated, these are symptoms of illness. Each one has a metabolic explanation but is also just a feeling. The more personally you take it, the bigger the story you build. Before you know it, thinking turns a runny nose into a severe virus, and a headache turns into a tumour. A feeling has turned into *The Feeling* now. And *The Feeling* has a more significant impact on metabolism than just a feeling.

There's nothing wrong with doing something in response to a feeling. You can lie down, eat, or take medication, but the situation escalates if the tides sweep over you. At the very least, you feel worse. Whenever you personalise a feeling and tighten around it, you're trying to control it in a way that makes it more unsatisfactory. If you let it be just a feeling, there will be less dissatisfaction. And because dissatisfaction impacts metabolism, it can increase metabolic stress, waste energy, and eventually make your illness worse, making you feel worse. When you feel worse, it's still just a feeling, but it's more than that because it's personal now.

Chapter 7 / What Does This Feeling Mean?

It's almost always true that what you think is wrong with you is more serious than what's wrong with you, and even when it isn't true, it's almost always better to assume it is. Yes, there are some exceptions to this rule, or at least to the first part, but still, it's almost always true. A big part of the reason is that people have gotten conditioned to respond to a feeling by thinking about it, and you know where that can lead!

When something is wrong with metabolism, the experts often say, "Nothing is wrong. It's just your imagination. Here, take this antidepressant". That's not particularly helpful, but it is a profitable business model. I'm not suggesting that health practitioners are dishonest or not experts. But plenty of uncertainty is inherent in the diagnosis and treatment of illness. Unfortunately, some might take advantage of that.

Regardless, health practitioners get told the "right way" to treat various ailments. Customers, sorry, I mean patients, love a cookie-cutter solution, so it's a perfect match. There's no shortage of patients because all it takes is for a painful or unpleasant feeling or sensation to arise and for some layers to get laid upon it. Many people want to know, "What does this feeling mean?"

People want an answer, but the answer is that there is no one single answer. What a feeling means biologically speaking depends on various things and is open to a lot of interpretation. And how a feeling plays out depends significantly on individual habitual reaction patterns rather than on a unique reason a feeling is there. So even if you knew the exact conditions that caused a feeling to arise and the actual changes required to make it disappear, how you react to it changes that.

And then, these habitual reaction patterns to a particular kind of feeling are strengthened by repetition. That's how they first became habitual. Plus, success bolsters them. You react a specific way to a sensation, and the situation improves, so the reaction is what caused the improvement.

Say a feeling that feels like fear arises. You don't like it, and there's tension. And you have a habit of thinking specific thoughts when it appears. You think about why the fear exists, why you don't like it, and what might happen. And how much you want it to go away. And if the fear subsides, you think that the reaction solved the problem of the fear because the fear went away. But it's an illusion or a delusion. It's not that you can't ever act. Talk to someone. Go for a walk. Take some medication if you need to. If you cut yourself, you get a bandage. It's not about that. How you feel is one thing, but *how you feel about how you feel* and beyond is another thing altogether. And this also drives the kind of actions you take.

When you tense up around a feeling you don't like, it can encourage a world of thinking, and you often barely notice you're thinking. You get so immersed in it that you hardly even realise it's happening. Next time a feeling of fear pops up if the same reaction gets set in motion, now it's heading in the direction of becoming a chronic reaction. Once again, it's not thinking per se that is harmful. For example, there's nothing wrong with thinking of ways to deal with fear.

Improving metabolism can reduce how much fear you feel. But the story you build around a feeling about what it means every time it arises can be the thing that ensures that it keeps appearing. "My fear", "my metabolic issues", "my bad experiences", "my demise". It's a self-defence reaction. But it's a reaction that usually doesn't make you safer, braver, healthier, or happier. And it doesn't end with stories. It is the stuff that emotions get made of. The more personal the story gets, the closer you get to the addition of emotion.

You are more than your emotions also. And although you don't control them personally, they don't just pop out of thin air for no reason. Emotions are the next layer that comes off of the previous layers. So now, *The Feeling* is even more significant and potentially more destructive. Emotion is still just a feeling, but it is powerful with a lot of habit-forming capability. For example, the more an emotion arises in response to a specific sensation, the more likely it will appear again next time. Then the meaning you give a feeling gets proven accurate, but it's a self-fulfilling prophecy. Before you know it, fear turns into anxiety; at some point, it can become panic.

And yet all it is is a feeling with layers added to it. But it's a more intense feeling that causes more suffering and significantly impacts metabolism. And all this is because you want to feel the way you want. But you're going about it the wrong way. As someone wise once said, "Don't be careful; you might hurt yourself".

Chapter 8 / You Can't Think Away A Feeling

When a feeling or sensation arises, the mind does what it does best. The mind thinks. Because it thinks thinking can fix whatever it thinks needs to get fixed about a feeling. The mind doesn't realise that you can't use thinking to make a feeling feel how you want it to feel. But you can use thinking to create more dissatisfaction and tension. And that leads to more thought and feeling. So it's not that thoughts are the enemy and must get eliminated. On the contrary, that way of thinking leads to even more thinking, dissatisfaction and tension, and eventually unhappiness. It's what you might call "mental proliferation".

> *What one feels, that one perceives and thinks about. What one thinks about, that one mentally proliferates. With what one has mentally proliferated as the source, perceptions and notions tinged by mental proliferation beset a man with respect to past, future, and present mind-objects cognizable through the mind* (Majjhima Nikāya 18. Madhupindika Sutta)

So what's the difference between thinking and wrong thinking or mental proliferation? There's never anything inherently wrong with thinking. But, in any case, it's not something you have control over or can stop. When a feeling arises, you take it personally if you don't like it and want it gone. That immediately sets off the automatic, unconscious, repetitive mind chatter that gets used to build the personal story about why you don't like it and want it gone. And what you believe it will do to you if it stays.

The personal story makes the "tides of conceiving" sweep over you. One way it does that is with emotion because emotion adds power and intensity to *The Feeling*. Mental proliferation or repetitive circular thinking is analogous to uncontrolled growth without differentiation of cancer. A cancer tumour is a self-defence mechanism against stress, but eventually, the defence becomes the stress.

When you can meet stress, it is called eustress; when you cannot, it becomes distress. It is not stress that is the problem. And it is not sensations, thoughts, or emotions that are the problem. It is the reaction or response that determines what they become. The reaction is an attempt to deal with the stress. Still, it often multiplies the stress, which can damage metabolism. When a feeling turns into *The Feeling*, that's another version of stress turning into distress. Not everyone gets harmed the same way by a certain kind of stress. The "perfect diet" doesn't work as well for everyone. Once you can recognize when and how layers get added to a feeling, you're witnessing the process that amplifies the impact of stress. It's easy to see that it's unnecessary.

Once you start dealing with a feeling with thinking, you open up a bottomless pit. The more you try to fix it, the bigger *The Feeling* gets. The bigger *The Feeling* becomes, the more stressful the stress becomes. And then the more likely it leads to issues with metabolism and unhappiness. Turning stress into distress makes it worse and interferes with metabolic energy systems. Therefore *The Feeling* wastes energy unnecessarily.

You can't think a feeling away. But there is another way. You can learn how to "unthink it".

Chapter 9 / Three "Noble" Metabolic Truths

If the Buddha returned today, he'd need to help people feel better and be happier even more than he did when he was here. So these are some things he'd say concerning metabolic health.

The first thing he'd say is that even if you figure out the perfect diet and lifestyle, there will always be things that can cause an unpleasant sensation to arise or make a good feeling disappear. But it's just a feeling, he'd say. And a feeling or sensation isn't the cause of unhappiness or suffering. Instead, the immediate, automatic, habitual reactions (the layers added to a feeling turning it into *The Feeling*) make all the difference.

Once you know this and learn what to do about it, a feeling can go back to being just a feeling, and you'll probably be happier and healthier. It's as simple as that, even if it isn't always easy, especially in the beginning.

> *Now this, bhikkhus, is the noble truth of the cessation of suffering: it is the remainderless fading away and cessation of that same craving, the giving up and relinquishing of it, freedom from it, nonreliance on it.* (SN 56:11 Dhammacakkappavattanasutta)

You can't stop a bad feeling from happening or make a good one stay, and that's basically what the mind is trying to do, using control. So what can you do? First, you must recognise that how you feel can be more than just how you feel. It can have *how you feel about how you feel, what you think about how you feel* in it, and more.

In one sense, when you have pain or feel ill, that is your reality. But it isn't your ultimate or fixed reality. It's a continuously fluctuating reality, so calling it an illness can be misleading. You don't like how you feel until you do again. That's all. I'm not suggesting there are no health emergencies. Still, it's fair to say that most suffering and unhappiness come not from health emergencies but from reactions and stories added to a feeling. So have a look for yourself.

Reactions and stories are illusory. They are not the truth. And even during a genuine health emergency, how you react and the story you tell in your head impacts outcomes. Of course, seeing things this way is far from easy when you're in a crisis. But practising with the little things is something you can do right now. Even if a feeling has become a part of your identity and you always react roughly the same way, adding layers to it, that doesn't mean it's how it has to be or how it is. If you notice that you're doing it, you can step back and look. Then you can take your attention off the thoughts and emotions to see what's underneath. Don't try to make the thoughts and emotions go away. Just look to see if you can see what's driving them. It is the beginning of understanding.

You are suffering, you feel unhappy, you feel pain, you feel anxiety. But it would help if you saw what's genuinely causing this. So if you look behind thinking and emotion and notice the tension in the mind-body, you see how you react to a feeling. The tension interferes with the flow of a sensation. It's an instinctive defensive reaction to wanting less or more of it and drives all the subsequent layers.

Pain or illness (mental or physical) are metabolic issues, and they get influenced by nervous system function, which gets influenced by an individual's particular history. So you create pathways over time. How they get made depends a lot on reactions to stress. Of course, nutrition and lifestyle are both factors, but how you respond to a feeling can override all that and change how you meet stress. Metabolically speaking, reacting to a tense feeling (followed by the other layers) is tantamount to interfering with metabolism flow. Allowing a sensation to run its course without adding layers is equivalent to meeting stress with the appropriate energy to handle it properly. That's a healthy metabolism.

If the Buddha were here now, he'd tell you to deal with stress by letting the stress-energy flow through without adding unnecessary interference. The Buddha would say to you that you must take your attention off the story and emotions to see the *craving* underneath so you can release the tension. It's called letting go. When you let go and release tension, you allow metabolic energy to flow and immediately feel relief. That's how it works, so once you realise it, you know how suffering and unhappiness get created on top of a feeling.

The more you practice letting go, the better you will see where the tension is. So the more opportunities you have to release it, the more relief you will experience. Releasing tension is the same as relaxing, and relaxation brings relief. Cultivating the ability to experience relief is the antidote to *The Feeling*. It's also how you divert metabolic pathways towards improved energy flow rather than the habit of going into a stress response. Stress interferes with energy flow, and relaxation promotes energy flow. Energy flow protects against stress and increases the ability to relax. It is the way.

You don't have to put a feeling right to feel better. Your natural state is unimpeded energy flow. So you only need to learn how to stop adding layers, and then how you feel will change. It doesn't sound like much, but it's the most important realisation.

The end of Part 1.

Part Two Dealing With The Feeling

Chapter 10 / All Pain Is Not Suffering

What do you do when you're in the middle of a crisis of feeling unwell, anxiety, depression, pain in the body, or any overwhelming feeling? First, you have to recognise what's happening. Otherwise, all bets are off. Thankfully the more you practice seeing when layers start adding to a feeling, the easier it gets to practice taking your attention off them. And the more you do that, the more likely you are to be able to do it next time, maybe even a little faster.

You take your attention off the thoughts and emotions, expanding a feeling, turning it into *The Feeling*. You don't have to do anything to them. When you stop focusing on them, you'll be able to see the tension in the mind-body better and relax it or allow it to flow through.

If you relax the tension, you might notice a feeling behind it. It usually has a tone or texture, although you won't be able to say what kind of feeling it is. It either feels unpleasant or pleasant. It's what leads to the *craving* reaction. It's how this whole mess began in the first place.

But now that you've relaxed a bit of your hold on it, just a feeling can start to burn itself out. In the burning, you might feel energy transforming or transmuting into the energy of relief. The energy of relief is a higher form of metabolic energy flow, which can change the state of metabolism and protect against stress. A feeling of relief is just a feeling that isn't being hindered or suppressed. So it's a more truthful free-flowing energy because there's less interference with its flow.

A painful or unpleasant feeling is not that different from a feeling of relief. When it arises, it doesn't equate to suffering. It's only a feeling with a slightly unsatisfactory tone. But once you react to it by trying to control it and adding a story, it can lead to disproportionate suffering and unhappiness. It doesn't have to be like this.

> *When one feels a painful feeling, one understands: 'I feel a painful feeling.' ...If he feels a painful feeling, he understands: 'It is impermanent; there is no holding to it; there is no delight in it.' ...if he feels a painful feeling, he feels it detached; For this...is the supreme noble wisdom, namely, the knowledge of the destruction of all suffering.* (Majjhima Nikāya 140. The Exposition of the Elements)

Noticing that a painful feeling has arisen can be the anchor for remembering to let the energy flow without adding any layers. When you see a painful feeling as just a pain, it's no longer your painful feeling. So it no longer bothers you the way it would with adding the personal story. But the tiniest of sensations, when connected to the story of "my pain", can trigger a reaction of adding layers, causing a lot of suffering. Personalisation is at the heart of craving, but you are more than your pain.

Every feeling is a form of metabolic energy. So if you interfere with energy flow, you interfere with metabolism, which has consequences. For example, you inhibit digestion and cannot fully utilise the best nutrition. At any point, if you allow a feeling to flow better or try to control it less, it will make you suffer less. When you try to control a feeling you don't like, you're trying to avoid an experience you don't like, making the experience worse. So avoiding suffering hides the truth and turns into the cause of suffering.

How you feel about how you feel turns just a feeling into a feeling causing suffering and unhappiness. You produce suffering and unhappiness out of an attempt to control energy flow. It isn't the inevitable result of the arising of a painful feeling. But a sensation can go from being just a feeling to *The Feeling* rapidly; you can easily mistake it for the cause of the suffering or the unhappiness that comes after it.

Suppressed energy is energy inadequately metabolised. In other words, suppressed energy is energy not processed fully. Instead, it leaves a residue that causes unnecessary metabolic interference. So it burns differently if a feeling is fully experienced, even if it is still painful, minus the added layers. It passes through without leaving as much of a trace. It feels different. It feels natural.

Chapter 11 / Fix Your Energy Fix Your Thyroid

Your energy system is only your energy system in a relative sense. So in another way, it isn't really "yours". Or you might say, "you are your energy system". Saying it these ways probably doesn't do justice to it, but for the sake of communication, it'll have to do for now.

Too much stress interferes with thyroid energy system metabolism. When you inhibit energy system metabolism, things often don't feel great. When things don't feel great, you suffer more and are less happy. So in one sense, it has to be that way. And in another altogether different sense, it doesn't have to be that way.

Metabolic issues are a fact of life, and that will never change. Thyroid function is not in your control. There are so many things that impact thyroid metabolism that you have no control over. However, it means that how you feel is going to change. If you want to control thyroid function, the best thing to do is to eliminate as many things as possible that interfere with energy metabolism. Then you can include more of what assists with energy metabolism. Diet and lifestyle are factors here, but the most important thing to eliminate is control itself. Only you can't do that with more control.

Nothing interferes with energy metabolism faster than control. Even the PUFAs and their breakdown products can't compete. The control reaction immediately interferes with energy flow. It is stress, by definition. The control reaction (or *craving*) is a push/pull reaction (shifting between liking and disliking how you feel) combined with tension or contraction. Sometimes it is necessary for self-protection, but more often than not, it's completely unnecessary.

Every time you notice it and relax it, you improve energy flow. You're improving energy metabolism. You're burning fuel more optimally and leaving behind less residue. It's like the difference between thyroid metabolism and stress metabolism. Too much stress can interfere with oxidative metabolism turning sugar into lactic acid instead of carbon dioxide. It is the incomplete burning of fuel.

Stress interferes with the ability of cells to relax and promotes an excited state that produces energy less optimally. Stress creates tension, which creates more stress and interference with energy flow. Overexcitation impedes the ability to relax, and anything that promotes relaxation promotes energy metabolism.

There's a direct relationship between digestion and mental stability issues involving substances that rise under stress and thyroid suppression, including serotonin, nitric oxide, lactic acid and bacterial endotoxin. Eating in a way that promotes digestion reduces exposure to bacterial endotoxin, serotonin, and other stress substances, improving mental stability, mood, and thyroid function. Psychological improvement also feeds back into overall energy metabolism improvement. Unfortunately, all this is also true in reverse, resulting in a downward spiralling thyroid energy system with worsening stress reactivity.

When stress is high, and you don't feel good, the control reaction (*craving*) leads to more control involving thinking and emotion. But unfortunately, it immediately inhibits digestion and impacts overall thyroid function.

You can do lots of the right things to fix thyroid energy metabolism and still interfere with metabolism regularly or continuously. It is often unseen processes driven by liking and disliking a feeling that makes up *how you feel about how you feel* and the other layers. They can cause unlimited metabolic interference, plus lots of suffering and unhappiness.

With awareness of these processes, combined with a practice of removing attention from the thinking/emotion storyline plus the release of tension in the mind-body, metabolic issues can head in the direction of being just a feeling. The more you practice observing these processes and stop taking them personally, the more subtle tensions you'll see, increasing your ability to relax and untrap "blocked" energy. You will begin to see you are more than your thoughts and emotions.

You don't want to hyper-focus on just a feeling, either, because that's what makes it grow. So please stop trying to make it go away. Allow it to go away naturally. The relief that arises from the relaxation of tension feels very good. So you can put your awareness in that general direction. But don't try to control it or try to make it stay. It never really went anywhere.

Chapter 12 / Imperfect Perfect Health

My yoga teacher, James, liked to say "80% Perfect"; it was usually the perfect time to get reminded. Nothing gets in the way of attaining perfection faster than a desire to achieve perfection. That's especially true when it comes to health. And no small part because there's no such thing as "perfect health". Although you might say, health is always perfectly imperfect.

Metabolism does not exist in a vacuum. It is not constant. Instead, it is constantly in flux. And the desire for health to be perfect interferes with the natural flow of things. Attaining perfect health is just a concept. Health issues are a daily part of life, consisting of ongoing interferences with energy flow and equilibrium. The tension plus other layers that follow from the reaction to a feeling create the opposite of a relaxed state, and nothing describes perfect health better than a relaxed state.

You can judge metabolism according to the ability to deal with stress and then return to a state of relaxation. For example, the Achilles tendon reflex test is an effective way to assess thyroid function. This test measures the ability to tense up and return to a state of relaxation. Generally speaking, the faster that occurs, the better thyroid metabolism.

But there is another way to achieve perfection, and this other kind of perfection does not require metabolism to be perfect. Lucky because striving to attain metabolic perfection is unlikely to lead to perfection. You can only achieve perfection by doing the opposite regularly. So you have to practice being unattached, which is a term that has received bad press unfairly. Absolute perfection comes from unattachment. Being unattached prevents a lot of suffering and unhappiness.

When you are unattached, a painful or unpleasant feeling will still arise. However, it will pass through you without the addition of unnecessary layers. That is perfection. All you have to do is notice when you are attached and stop. Simple, not always easy.

You are attached when a feeling arises that you don't like and want to go away and tense up around it. When more layers get added, you are more attached. That's alright because you can practice non-attachment when you become aware of this. Just take your attention away from thoughts and emotions and relax the underlying tension. But don't try too hard because that will cause more attachment. Perfectionism is attachment, and it prevents the attainment of perfection.

Even if you relax tension, you won't necessarily feel good immediately. Removing your attention from thinking and emotion is not intended to make it disappear. *The Feeling* is not the enemy and doesn't need to be crushed down or pushed away. Using force won't make you feel better, not for long anyway. The more you can relax when a feeling arises, the less attached you are to it, and then the less it is part of the personal story of "your health" or "your happiness". Attachment is taking it personally.

> *Many people imagine that every spiritual master has, or should have, the health and strength of a Sandow. The*

> *assumption is unfounded. A sickly body does not indicate that a guru is not in touch with divine powers, any more than lifelong health necessarily indicates an inner illumination* (Autobiography Of A Yogi, Paramahansa Yogananda).

There's nothing wrong with thinking or emotion. But dissatisfaction with a feeling arises out of the distortion of a feeling. It is trapped energy that is unable to express itself freely. When energy flows freely, dissatisfaction, tension, and unhelpful thoughts and emotions dissipate.

Good and bad states are always coming and going. If you are alive, it cannot be any other way. Stress is a part of life, and thyroid function fluctuates. It would feel great to have perfect metabolic health, but it's a fantasy. How you respond to a feeling (good or bad) determines how much you suffer and how happy you are, not the arising feeling itself. When you allow a feeling to be just a feeling, it becomes a form of therapy.

And the less attached you are to a feeling, the less it interferes with metabolism because a relaxed, happy state is never far away. It is always there; it only gets temporarily hidden. So it's the art of improving health and happiness without trying to improve health and happiness.

Health is good for happiness, and happiness is good for health. But, unfortunately, dissatisfaction and tension get in the way, especially if you try to make a feeling go away or stay. So what you need is what the Buddha referred to as equanimity. It's a mind-body that takes things as they come—no unnecessary interference.

Trying to achieve perfect health leads to suppression. You're trying to avoid feeling what you don't want to feel. But that turns a feeling into *The Feeling*, which does not promote perfect health. It sounds simplistic, but that's because it is simple. Being unattached is about feeling what you feel when you feel it. Perfectionism is about what you want or don't want to happen. You can't stop what happens when it happens. Still, you can take it less personally or seriously, leading to freedom from suffering and unhappiness.

A feeling will arise, will be fully metabolised, and will end. The more you can let go of your attachment to it, the more you will see that it is the attachment that causes so much suffering and unhappiness. And it can also interfere with metabolism and health. It certainly feels that way.

Chapter 13 / Replacing Pathways To Stress

Exposure to improperly met stress creates pathways that make turning on the stress reaction easier. These pathways are like rivers. The more they flow in a particular direction, the easier it becomes for them to flow in that direction and gain more momentum. If a feeling arises in the mind-body and you try to control it, you add layers that help create a stress pathway. Then, like a river, the next time a similar feeling arises, you're more likely to attempt to control it roughly the same way, reinforcing the pathway. That's forming a habit.

The tension created from *craving* (wanting less or more of a feeling) interferes with energy flow, suppressing the thyroid and promoting stress substances like adrenaline, cortisol, lactic acid and more. This reaction moves from "rest and digest" towards "fight or flight". You might not notice it initially, but reinforcing a stress pathway makes your stress system more dominant. If you add an attempt to control thinking and emotion, the stress becomes more noticeable. Eventually, the stress system can take charge.

Digestion is where you often notice the effects of a chronic stress response. The link between stressful thoughts and digestion is well known. However, how noticeable depends on the strength of metabolic stress/nervous system pathways. It sounds daunting, but it's an opportunity. Because just like you can create a path, you can uncreate one.

Stress is not something to get rid of because the attempt to get rid of it is what builds it in the first place. So striving to stop a stress pathway is what strengthens the stress pathway. So that's why people struggle to eliminate stress. It's because they're struggling. And stress doesn't need to be stopped. When stress arises, just seeing it creates some separation between it and the story of the stress. This separation makes the personal story less personal. Then it'll be easier to see and relax the tension you have layered on top of the stress.

Stress is the perfect reminder to relax the mind-body, and you might feel warm relief. It is what unimpeded energy metabolism feels like. It can be cultivated by staying out of the way and allowing the energy to move freely. It's how to replace a stress pathway. The more relief you feel, the more you create new paths that don't rely on stress. So you're building a new habit that responds to stress without adding more. Like a river with a small amount of water flowing off the main path, the new way is barely noticeable initially. Still, if it can grow, the whole river can eventually flow in a new direction. Then, you don't need to stop anything. But you do have to practice, or else the little streams might not grow enough to move away from the momentum-increasing existing stress pathways. And practice means taking advantage of when you notice you have gone into stress. It redirects your attention away from the stress story to "bring relaxation" to the tension in the mind-body. It is how you make a new habit. Or, to be more accurate, it is how you become more aware of your natural state.

The warm relief when tension is relaxed and energy metabolism is improved relates to the feeling of loving-kindness. The Buddha, the world's most famous meditation teacher, recommended bringing it up. When it arises, you can place your awareness lightly on it, slowly cultivating it. It's how you gradually replace a pathway to stress, enabling energy flow and protecting against suffering and unhappiness. Just ensure you don't get too attached to the excellent feeling because that will bring the tension and all the other layers, and the whole thing will sneak in again through the back door.

Chapter 14 / Feed Metabolism Not Stress

What you feed metabolism impacts the way metabolism functions. So it's not just about what you put in your mouth; in a sense, it's still about eating. Your metabolism is eating even if you haven't put food in your mouth. Now it's eating what you have stored in the body and eating the body. So the makeup of the body becomes the thing that impacts how metabolism functions.

It can go as far as determining whether you're in a constant state of stress or whether you're working with thyroid energy metabolism. Most people are somewhere in between. It still has to do with what you eat because what you eat changes what you have stored in the body.

A pro-metabolic way of eating is one way to feed metabolism, not stress. And it's an effective way to protect against stress.

> *The yogi should eat nourishing, sweet foods mixed with milk. They should benefit the senses and stimulate the functions* (Yoga Swami Svatmarama. Hatha Yoga Pradipika).

Certain foods are well-named as pro-metabolic, and other foods are not so much. It isn't a black-and-white thing because metabolism is never black-and-white. But it isn't random, either, far from it. Logical and testable arguments exist in favour of some ingredients over others. And there's been a lot of testing.

Even though this book does not explore the impact of pro-metabolic eating on metabolism, it is relevant to the subject. It's particularly relevant concerning what happens to metabolism when excess stress occurs. Stress promotes the release of free fatty acids from storage and into the bloodstream. Polyunsaturated free fatty acids (from a diet high in PUFAs) damage thyroid function and promote chronic stress.

Stressful thinking and emotion powerfully promote biochemical stress and free fatty acid release. It's easy to demonstrate. Start thinking about something worrying and watch what happens. You can feel the adrenaline rising, and guess what that means! It means increasing exposure to free fatty acids.

When fat released into circulation is high in PUFAs, damage to energy metabolism is far more significant. In addition, exposure to the substances that promote chronic stress (like estrogen, nitric oxide, serotonin, bacterial endotoxin and cortisol) increases. Increased stress substance exposure promotes tension and repetitive circular thinking and emotion. Mental stress (even without high exposure to PUFAs) increases metabolic demands and shifts metabolism away from digestion, promoting more biochemical stress.

Sweet foods are pro-metabolism and anti-stress because they fuel the thyroid and help keep the stress substances at bay. They feed metabolism, not stress, which means they help metabolism meet stress with sufficient energy. They promote metabolic equilibrium. But you can also be in balance when metabolism is not. That's equanimity.

Metabolic equilibrium is about how you feel. Equanimity is more about *how you feel about how you feel*. If you allow a feeling to be just a feeling, it doesn't matter what feeling it is. So you're feeding metabolism, not stress, even if it's a stressful feeling. On the other hand, suppose you have developed the habit of responding to a sensation arising with dissatisfaction and tension (*craving*). In that case, you feed stress even if your metabolism functions well.

A stressed metabolism already promotes tension over relaxation. It increases exposure to stressful thoughts and emotions, but *how you feel about how you feel* and *what you think about how you feel* have a multiplying effect. So you're feeding stress, and the more you do it, the stronger the pathways to stress, and then the less you can fix it by eating the right food or having the proper lifestyle.

Equanimity in the face of stress means choosing a different response whenever you notice that you are reacting with a stress habit. That's how you start to unlearn a stress habit and create a pathway away from suffering towards your true nature, happiness. But, again, the circumstances are not the issue here.

You do not deny stress, suppress emotions, or push a painful feeling away. Instead, you're doing the opposite. It is about allowing a feeling to be there as just a feeling, without the need to focus on it, while it burns itself out with little interference. You're creating separation so that you can see a feeling less personally. If it isn't personal, it's just a feeling, not *The Feeling*.

Whenever you can bring relaxation to the tension in the mind-body, you're allowing for a complete metabolising of the energy in a feeling behind the tension. So that brings up a warm sense of relief. It's known as transmutation. It's an uncovering. The trapped energy of stress gets freed to flow as positive metabolic energy, feeding metabolic healing. So an unattached feeling has the potential to heal long-term metabolic stress. But don't be too focused on achieving that outcome, or it will become more of the same thing that leads to where you are.

Chapter 15 / PTSDissipation

PTSD stands for Post Traumatic Stress Disorder, which is a pretty fair description. However, I also think the name says more about what PTSD is than lots of people realise. Something traumatic (or many traumatic things) happened to you, producing a stress response. The stress response was big enough or went on for long enough to cause your stress response system to become disordered (if it wasn't already).

A disordered stress response system promotes a stress response that is no longer objectively appropriate regarding circumstances. For example, it's too intense, stays around for too long, or happens out of the blue for seemingly no apparent reason.

The DSM-5 criteria for diagnosis of PTSD require direct or indirect exposure to a traumatic event, followed by symptoms from four categories: intrusion, avoidance, negative changes in thoughts and mood, and changes in arousal and reactivity. Something traumatic happens, and chronic stress symptoms follow it. It isn't rocket science, although neither is all rocket science.

There isn't a tremendous amount of certainty in diagnosing PTSD (or bipolar and schizophrenia), and there is no shortage of theories regarding the metabolic/biochemical milieu that promotes and goes with it. That's because stress can lead to a variety of symptoms and a variety of metabolic changes. So sometimes, what sounds like an opposing metabolic scenario is just another expression of what can happen due to exposure to excessive or chronic stress. For example, are cortisol levels too high or too low in PTSD? You can confirm both, resulting from excessive and ongoing stress exposure.

High cortisol can be a response to unmet stress, and low cortisol can result from even more unmet stress. Low cortisol can be from the stress that has been going on for a long time, often together with low thyroid and low cholesterol and various nutritional deficiencies. Whether cortisol is too high or too low, reducing stress exposure and increasing metabolic resilience to stress is the way.

Hyper-reactivity to stress reinforces the pathways that lead to PTSD. So every time a feeling arises, and you react to it with the addition of dissatisfaction and tension and all the rest, you are reinforcing the pathways that promote hyper-reactivity. PTSD is a system in an overexcited state, responding with stress to every stress, regardless of whether it is stressful or not. The habit of responding to uncomfortable energy with stress has become entrenched. This energy can be a sensation, memory, mood, or thought about the future. It doesn't matter. It all gets taken personally as part of the story of "My PTSD". It produces *The Feeling* rapidly thanks to the fuel that comes from attachment. The automatic trying to make a feeling go away is what can make it more powerful, intense, overwhelming and metabolically interfering.

The objective severity of the original trauma is not what determines whether PTSD will be the result. Many people are diagnosed with PTSD without experiencing extreme trauma. Lots of small stresses can do it. Also, people face terrible conditions for long periods without getting PTSD. It is partly due to metabolic variation. But *how you feel about how you feel* and all the other layers that make up *The Feeling* do not require extreme trauma to thrive. The layers create trauma for you, and the stress pathways get created from that. So when *The Feeling* grows, a personal story grows, justifying how it feels.

Although PTSD isn't a single-factor issue, hyper-responsiveness to a feeling arising drives the symptoms. They are difficult to experience, see past, and calm when you're in the middle of experiencing them. A pro-metabolic (sattvic) diet and lifestyle make it easier to look at things with equanimity so that you can practise dealing with *The Feeling* when you see it begin to grow.

The easiest way to improve PTSD is one feeling at a time, one reaction at a time. It can gradually dissipate the stress reaction pathways and create a new habitual healing response; yes, it's cumulative in either direction. And every time you get lost in *The Feeling* and notice that you're lost, you're no longer lost.

Then you can look for some tension and dissatisfaction. And you can bring some relaxation to the situation and get some relief. You don't have to stop anything or make anything go away. The relaxed state was always there. You're just looking in a new direction and then allowing a feeling to flow, dissipating trapped energy every time you see an opportunity. So you're taking it one stress reaction at a time.

Chapter 16 / Look, Let Go, Digest

Looking more closely won't automatically make you an expert at seeing a feeling, thought, emotion, or tension arise and immediately allow it to pass freely through. I'm no expert yet, but it doesn't matter. What matters is once you start noticing these processes that have always been happening without you noticing, it's hard to go back to not seeing them again.

It's like what happens when you learn new eating methods that improve digestion and metabolism, and then the impact is more pronounced after a while if you eat something you used to eat but no longer eat. It's not a foolproof test for the healthiness of food. Still, when it comes to *The Feeling*, once you know how to unhook your attention and relax the tension, it's hard to ignore how much it improves your overall state.

As I said, you won't catch it every time, and that's alright. It happens very quickly and stealthily. Wanting to see it every time is more perfectionism; you know where that leads! But you will start to see the process happening more the more you see it. That's how momentum works. When you see a feeling, you have a choice to make. Either allow it to be just a feeling or take it personally and try to control it. Either you hold on, or you let go.

Letting go doesn't mean you stop anything or make anything go away. You don't have to "empty your mind" or stare at a candle. And there's nothing to fix. You got caught in a loop, and now you aren't, even if the loop is still running its course. Letting go means you stop adding fuel to it. It will burn out when it burns out. If you don't feel good, the habit is to try to influence it with your mind because you don't like it. You don't want to let it be what it is. You want to resist it, but that creates tension, and tension prevents you from feeling good. So the less strain, the better you feel.

> *Let it be, let it be*
> *Let it be, yeah, let it be*
> *Oh, there will be an answer Let it be*
> *Let it be, let it be*
> *Let it be, yeah, let it be Whisper words of wisdom Let it be* (The Beatles)

Nutrition is vital for digestion because it fuels metabolism, and digestion improves if metabolism improves. Unfortunately, toxins build up in the intestines when you consume many anti-metabolic and difficult-to-digest foods. Then any time you get exposed to stress and intestinal barrier function inhibition, more toxins pass through to the liver, adding to the stress.

The anti-metabolic PUFAs interfere with digestion and promote metabolic stress and inflammation. In addition, if you eat them regularly, they get stored in tissue over time, making the consequences of stress more severe. A pro-metabolic diet can protect you from stress damage and improve healing and recovery potential. But everything to do with metabolism works better when you practice looking, letting go, and relaxing the tension.

When you take a feeling personally and try to control it, energy diverts away from essential metabolic functions like digestion. The pathways to stress and suboptimal digestion strengthen if you do this often. Digestive dysfunction becomes a habit. Stress gets momentum behind it. And then perfect nutrition is no longer perfect. The better you notice the *craving* reaction and relax, the more protected you are from difficult-to-digest anti-metabolic foods. Because when you relax tension, you improve energy flow, making imperfect nutrition less imperfect. Or, to put it differently, it will make the consequences of poor nutrition less consequential.

Just try not to forget that relaxing tension is not something you force. The force turns it back into stress. It helps to see a rising feeling like a ball resting in the palm of your hand. If you squeeze it tightly, you waste energy and create tension. If you open your hand and let it rest in your palm, you're letting go and relaxing. You're also resting and digesting. Being able to relax the tension in the mind-body has many unintended benefits. Combining a sattvic diet with a sattvic mind creates a powerful synergy.

Looking inside, letting go and relaxing the tension in the mind-body is not about control. It's about releasing it, uncovering what is always there. So you're going with the flow, which powerfully influences how you feel. And if it doesn't, at the very least, it will powerfully influence *how you feel about how you feel*. And that feels good.

Chapter 17 / Everybody Needs Attention

Attention is a fact of life; everybody needs it and has it. You can't get rid of it, even if you want to. Your attention has to go somewhere, and where it goes impacts how you feel in multiple ways. One problem with attention is that it's easier to keep it on a painful or uncomfortable, or unpleasant feeling than it is to keep it on a good one. That's because it's a feeling you don't like. You want it to go away, and deep down, you believe keeping your attention on it will do something to help make it go away and help bring back a feeling you do like.

Because you look at it with dissatisfaction, this brings tension. Then you think about your dissatisfaction, making it more personal and significant. You think about what you think it is, why it's there, why you don't want it, what will happen if it stays, what if it gets worse, and so on. All this makes you feel worse. But even though you feel worse, part of you thinks keeping your attention on it and thinking about it helps. Maybe because you've always done that, it got you this far. So what to do? Keep looking at it and thinking about it. But, no, I'm just kidding, don't do that!

It's a bit more complicated, but this sums up what drives repetitive thinking and lots of the things that come with it. Deep down, there's a belief it's helping. And perhaps it is helping in a way, but that's a dangerous belief because it makes it much harder to stop. Because you think the situation would be worse if you weren't doing all that.

Also, the more your attention goes where it goes, the easier it is to go there again. So that's momentum or pathway creation. And it influences metabolism, which affects the kind of feeling that arises. So it can promote a vicious circle. When you focus on a feeling you don't like, you multiply its power and increase how long it stays. It becomes part of your personal story, meaning you get attached to it.

You can be attached to a good feeling too. You want more of it and don't want it to go away. It's the other side of the coin. The issue is attachment, not a feeling or whether it's bad or good. The problem is your relationship with it—the desire not to feel bad or to keep feeling good leads to the same place. Trying to make a feeling you like to stick around is usually enough to make it not stick around.

Most people get more practice reacting to a bad feeling. But either way, it can still become part of your story of dissatisfaction. It can be a story about how the opposite of what you want to happen always happens, and it can go on like that for decades unless you see the trick. It's not about faking how you feel or pretending to like a feeling you don't like. That's just more *craving*. How you feel is how you feel. It's a feeling. But *how you feel about how you feel* adds personal meaning to it, and that meaning is only relatively accurate at best. So a feeling arises, and even when it's just a mild sensation, the relevant story reloads, and the "tides of conceiving" start to wash over you.

A sensation with the addition of *craving* can easily lead to anxiety or depression, or even panic. And that makes

The Feeling grow more prominent, and the bigger it gets, the more you want to change how you feel. And if you don't know, you won't see the pattern even though it's repeating itself, and it's a self-fulfilling prophecy. You build your reasoning into the story that gets attached to a feeling. You don't see that it's just a feeling with layers. It gets constructed inside your attention, but one thing that never gets touched is your attention.

All this keeps recurring until a feeling can be just an impersonal feeling. Then the energy can flow through with less resistance, eventually burning out completely. It's like the difference between eustress and distress, or stress that's met versus unmet stress. When you let a feeling be just a feeling, you feel it more fully. Then it doesn't leave a residue like sugar, turning into lactic acid. You're producing more carbon dioxide instead.

When a feeling can be just that, it doesn't matter as much what kind of feeling it is. So minus the layers, it's no longer noticeably good or bad. The aim isn't to make yourself feel good because you can't. You're just letting go of your hold on a feeling, allowing a warm sense of relief to arise. Then you can lightly rest your attention there. Please don't focus on it too hard or try to control anything. If you tread lightly, you'll see this relief feeling is a feeling that permanently resides underneath the interference with energy. It's your natural state. It feels warm, like thyroid metabolism and like friendliness.

Chapter 18 / Default To Happiness

It might sound like a strange idea that you can be happy for no reason because, for most people, it also sounds like a strange idea that you can be unhappy for no reason. That's because there's never any shortage of reasons to justify unhappiness. If you wait long enough, one of those reasons will pop into your mind or happen.

But another way to see this is that unhappiness is just a feeling. So the reasons that justify or explain why you feel bad are layered on top. These reasons make an unhappy feeling bigger and stronger, regardless of whether true or not. So it's how to create *The Feeling*.

Of course, bad things do happen. Something bad will happen eventually. And when it does, it doesn't feel good or easy. However, a feeling of unhappiness often comes up for no reason at all, and it can go away for similar unknown reasons. At least, that's how it looks.

Before an unhappy feeling becomes an emotion, it's just a sensation or feeling that arises that is open to interpretation. It's just trapped energy or metabolism interacting with the environment. It may start with a slightly unsatisfactory bent. Still, it gets interpreted, adding dislike, tension, thinking, and emotion, not necessarily in that order.

What happens after a feeling arises determines how unhappy you become. And that is only sometimes determined by the seriousness of the situation. There's no shortage of miserable people with life circumstances that are, objectively speaking, not so bad. And some other people who live under harsh conditions are more happy. So how do you explain that? The answer is it depends on whether you default to unhappiness or whether you default to happiness. Your default pathway is just a created habit. The only way to change this is to create a new one, one feeling at a time. And it's difficult at first because your default pathway has a lot of momentum.

A feeling or thought or emotion arises, and all you have to do is let it be without adding layers, but you don't like it and want it gone. It's just one moment, but it's tough to resist trying to control it. And when you do, you've just made it more difficult. It's like a mosquito bite. At first, it's just a little itchy. It doesn't feel that bad, but the temptation to scratch it is there. You don't like it, and you're trying to make it stop by itching it. You know how that usually works out.

Defaulting to happiness doesn't mean you only feel good things. It means you allow a feeling to pass through, even if it's unhappy. You see it for what it is. It's just a feeling. It doesn't arise with meaning already attached to it. Instead, you add a story around it, and that makes it less accurate, not more. And less genuine.

It was never your personal feeling, and you don't have to get rid of it. All you do is get out of its way. Relaxing the tension is part of getting out of its way. To relax, you just let go of your hold. Then a feeling you don't like will move through with less resistance, and a good one can come up sooner rather than later.

However, a good feeling can also strengthen a default to unhappiness because you like it and want it to stay. It's the same *craving* that has tension built into it. A good feeling can lead some people to fear happiness because it brings with it the prospect of leaving, which brings stress and dissatisfaction now and later. But true happiness cannot leave because it is your default state that gets covered up.

Defaulting to happiness doesn't mean making happiness arise and stay. It just means allowing a feeling to be there when it's there and not to be there when it isn't. True happiness is in the allowing; it is not a sensation, thought or emotion. But you can still enjoy a good feeling when it's available, and as long as you don't try too hard to make it stay, it will come back more often and last longer.

Chapter 19 / Relaxing Metabolic Craving

Trying to relax is like staring at one of those Magic Eye autostereograms from the 90s. When you try too hard to see the hidden image, you won't be able to see it. It makes people try harder to see it until it gives them a headache, and they give up, frustrated, possibly thinking there was no image to see in the first place.

The harder you stare at the 2D psychedelic pattern, the more difficult it gets. But if you look through the page, soften your gaze and stop trying (maybe go a little cross-eyed), you'll see a 3D image materialise and float off the page. Who'd have thought it was the trying preventing you from seeing it in the first place? It's the same with a feeling you don't like, don't try to get rid of it because that's what makes it feel not good—trying to get rid of it.

You're trying to eliminate it because you don't like it and think you can make it disappear. But there's another reality available. The 3D image you're not seeing. You can't see it because the layers on top are blinding you. You reacted to a feeling with dissatisfaction and tension, and you turned it into *The Feeling*. The more you resist it, the bigger it gets and the harder it is to fight, adding more resistance. Even so, all you have to do at any point is look past it. Then you'll see the actual picture, your naturally relaxed state. Wanting to control it morphed it into something unrecognisable. Like with the Magic Eye picture, once you see how it works, it's easier to do it next time.

Nothing has changed. It was always there.

> *The Great Way is not difficult for those who have no preferences. When love and hate are both absent everything becomes clear and undisguised. Make the smallest distinction, however, and heaven and earth are set infinitely apart. If you wish to see the truth then hold no opinion for or against. The struggle of what one likes and what one dislikes is the disease of the mind.* (Sengstan).

Your metabolism isn't yours. It's more like "you're metabolising". But when a feeling gets personalised, it becomes harder to see the actual state of metabolism. It becomes dysfunctional. But you aren't stuck with a feeling if it is just a feeling. Then it's easier for the metabolism to return to equilibrium. When it becomes *The Feeling*, it has stress built into it, keeping it going. The layers drive additional metabolic interference, like a downward spiralling vicious circle.

You can't control metabolism, but if a feeling is just a feeling, metabolism can metabolise with less in the way. So even if metabolic dysfunction persists, the less stress and tension added, the less suffering and unhappiness it brings.

The more you allow a feeling to be just that by relaxing your hold on it, the chances are you will get an improvement in metabolism. When you relax the *craving*, inhibiting metabolism, you're allowing the relief hidden underneath a feeling to arise. So it's like a hidden picture. Relaxing is not something you do. It's something you undo. You're releasing something already there; it's your natural state. It's what all sensations, thoughts, and emotions get made out of. You just let it flow, and it can grow. The warm feeling of relief has many incarnations, but we can call it uninhibited energy metabolism. The more it flows, the better it handles stress.

You "untense" the tension, but first, you have to know it's there, and you won't if you get caught in the layers. The issue is not on the surface of the picture. It won't matter how hard you try if your attention remains focused there. You won't be able to see what you need to see, hidden right in front of you. Happiness is the same. The more you search, the less available it is; but it's right here.

Chapter 20 / The Buddha's Metabolism

The Buddha tried all the ways available to figure out the best way to fix issues with the mind-body. Of course, these methods did not work how he hoped. But they led him to realise that adding stress to stress does not fix stress. In other words, you can't fix stress by pushing it away, suppressing it, or distracting yourself because all those things add more stress to stress or fail to deal with it.

The difference between a metabolism relying on backup stress systems and a metabolism relying on thyroid energy systems comes down to that point where stress meets metabolism. If metabolism can meet the stress demand, then it can be beneficial. If it can't, the stress systems kick in, and the situation is no longer optimal. Likewise, when you respond to a feeling with tension plus other layers, the result is a feeling not fully felt. That leaves a residue. It adds stress, just like suboptimally metabolised sugar.

On that note, something else The Buddha realised was that restrictive dieting and fasting aren't the way forward. It just leads to more stress, which adds stress to stress. That's why it's helpful to understand the fundamentals of pro-metabolic (sattvic) eating. It can help stabilise the mind-body to create a better environment for observing the processes of creating *The Feeling*. It helps to see them, to let them go.

But diet alone isn't enough to compensate for the habitual reaction of tension coming off an arising feeling. Even when the diet is close to optimal, interfering with the flow of a feeling can turn the perfect diet into the perfect storm.

Suppression is never optimal, which applies to metabolism and stress. It also applies to just a feeling arising in the mind-body. A pro-metabolic diet helps promote the metabolic equivalent of letting go and relaxing. In contrast, anti-metabolic eating promotes suppression of thyroid function. A healthy metabolism promotes relaxation, but being able to see and release tension in the mind-body can take metabolism to another level.

The Buddha figured out that trying to stop stress with stress, or "crush mind with mind", causes more stress and more mind. There is, however, a big difference between using thinking to fix problems caused by thinking and allowing thoughts to go wherever they flow and relaxing the tension fuelling them. Without the *craving*, thinking is just thinking. It can be helpful, but it isn't personal. And the *craving* gets driven by the identification with the story that hides your naturally relaxed state, equivalent to happiness.

The Buddha understood that how you deal with stress determines if stress is beneficial or harmful. He knew the difference between eustress and distress comes from how you meet stress. The mind-body functions best without interference because it is interference that drives dysfunction. Everything is in flow, so "having a disease" is more like the mind-body is "diseasing". Getting worse or getting better depends on momentum. However, there are ways to speed up momentum, and there are ways to slow it down.

You don't control metabolism, and you don't control whether or not you get sick. But you can allow metabolism to move toward improvement by no longer adding unnecessary friction. All you do is let metabolism be metabolism. It's the art of doing without doing, aka the art of undoing.

Chapter 21 / Cool Heat

All is burning. All is burning. But what is this all that is burning? And not only that, what kind of burning is the burning that is burning? What kind of burning do you want, and how does it compare to the burning you don't want? All burning is not made equal. Different kinds of burning create different kinds of heat. So it's essential to differentiate between them. There's damp heat and cool heat. There's overheating from dysfunction, and then there's the right amount of metabolic heat.

> *Bhikkhus, all is burning. And what is the all that is burning? The eye is burning, forms are burning, eye consciousness is burning, eye contact is burning, and whatever feeling arises with eye contact as condition-whether pleasant or painful, or neither-painful-nor-pleasant-that too is burning. Burning with what? Burning with the fire of lust, with the fire of hatred, with the fire of delusion; burning with birth, aging, and death; with sorrow, lamentation, pain, displeasure, and despair, I say.* (The Connected Discourses of The Buddha)

When energy gets fully burned, it creates a clean, cool heat. However, interference in the form of excess stress creates a damp, unclean heat that doesn't feel very good, especially if you compare the difference. Still, it's easy to confuse the two because metabolic heat production is good. So heat from stress can also be helpful, even though it is a source of problems. Like all things stress, it's good until it isn't.

People confuse a genuinely high metabolism with a "fast metabolism" fueled by stress. A metabolism that runs on stress is often overheated. It is hypothyroid, but it can look hyperthyroid. A high metabolism meets stress effectively with thyroid energy production. It burns fuel fully and produces a cool heat, or you might say it "hurries slowly". As a result, optimal metabolic function is relaxed even under pressure.

The burning that results from tension, dissatisfaction, and other layers of *The Feeling*, burns with "the fire of delusion". When you meet a feeling by taking it personally and tensing up, the true nature of that feeling is hidden, inhibiting the energy behind it. Partial burning produces damp heat and leaves a residue. It is suboptimal energy production. Each new layer adds interference, eventually promoting an over-excited inflamed mind-body. It's reflected metabolically as stress and cellular excitation. This kind of state promotes repetitive thinking, emotional dysregulation, chronic pain, anxiety, depression and metabolic illness in general.

Suppose you put pro-metabolic food into a dysregulated, over-excited, overheated system. In that case, you cannot utilise the metabolic value of that food because stress interferes directly with metabolism. Still, the metabolic consequences are more extreme in a blood sugar-dysregulated, waterlogged system laden with PUFAs and overloaded with iron and other inflammatory things.

Cellular excitation increases exponentially when the mind reacts with excitation to a body reacting with excitation. The damp heat produced as a result feels terrible, and the temptation is to do something about it. But, of course, there's nothing wrong with doing something, as long as what you do isn't just more of what you did to get here.

When *how you feel about how you feel* adds resistance to a feeling, a feeling doesn't get fully felt, which causes stress, tension and damp heat production. If thyroid function can meet stress, this promotes a relaxed cellular environment, which goes together with a relaxed mind. Both promote energy metabolism and healing. Cool heat is healing heat.

Stress is a fact of life. How you respond to a feeling determines how much suffering comes from it. Stress is more manageable if you allow a feeling to be just a feeling, minus the story of you and your stress. Bringing cool heat to dissatisfactory circumstances promotes relaxation and relief, and happiness, even under conditions that are not ideal. A feeling won't end until it ends, but now it doesn't have to escalate into *The Feeling*. Pain and discomfort are still there. A living metabolism can always bring a good or bad sensation. The personalisation of just a feeling brings on suffering and unhappiness.

Personalisation means liking and disliking and tension, aka *craving*. But not just liking or disliking; it has "the story of you" built into it. You think you can't be happy until you fix it, but *craving* separates you from your natural state: happiness. It produces a damp heat of resisted or inhibited energy flow.

The personalisation of a feeling is an avoidance technique. It's a diversion away from completely feeling a feeling. At best, it adds relatively true meaning, but it leads to feeling worse. It's dealing with stress, with the addition of more stress. It is not the way.

Chapter 22 / Making Your System Nervous

Few things stress your nervous system as much as mental/emotional distress. And few things can increase mental/emotional stress, like a distressed nervous system. For example, repetitive thinking and mental/emotional distress go hand in hand, and the nervous system responds to repetitive circular thinking very quickly. Circular thinking is a driver of metabolic stress and is almost always dysfunctional. Of course, it probably is always dysfunctional, but it's nice to leave some room for an exception here and there.

An overly stressed metabolism doesn't feel good, and a distressed nervous system doesn't, either. So it makes more sense when you know how much influence the nervous system has over metabolic function. The truth is all things to do with nervous system function, metabolism, and the mind-body are interconnected. So you don't want to have a dysregulated nervous system as much as you don't want to have a stressed metabolism. It is why repetitive thinking is a problem.

> *The nervous system is in control of metabolism to a great extent so you don't have to run five miles to shift over into that stress metabolism if your nervous system and emotional systems are very stressed* (Dr Ray Peat, PhD).

The irony is rumination attempts to fix a nervous or tense system. But instead, it does little except increase nervousness, tension, and rumination. Rumination is the mind attempting to make a painful or unpleasant feeling disappear. But it just creates a diversion or distraction. When a feeling like fear or anxiety arises, rumination builds a story that might as well be titled "How to avoid this feeling that I don't like".

But all the dissatisfaction with it and the tension coming from that make you dislike it even more. The mind thinks it's working out a solution, but all it's doing is creating a new and more significant problem. Rumination helps make your whole system nervous. It helps build a pathway making nervous system excitation the norm. And that means a stressed metabolism too. Then the best diet or the best lifestyle is far less beneficial.

It was common knowledge that eating is not good when anxious or stressed. And it's easy to see how nervousness impacts digestion, appetite, and enjoyment of food. But, of course, you can eat foods that help stop anxiety and stress, and it's natural to want to stop them. But it's also the wanting to stop it that can stop it from stopping because wanting increases rumination.

Repetitive thinking can promote actions that also make *The Feeling* grow. You think you're doing what needs doing, but you need to see what's making *The Feeling* grow in the first place. When you are off fixing it, you're likely to miss that. It doesn't mean what you decided to do was wrong or wouldn't be able to help. Still, very often, it's a bandaid solution, and you fail to address the real cause of the escalation of *The Feeling*. If you feel like you've tried all the ways to feel better and still don't feel the way you want, you may be missing something subtle that's right there whenever you don't feel the way you want to feel. And what it is, is wanting to feel different.

You see a feeling as more than just a feeling. You see it as your feeling, meaning it must get controlled, or it will take over. But what you need is to uncontrol it. You need to disidentify with it or disassociate from it. But, again, it's just a feeling, and identifying with it adds tension, interfering with its flow and separating it from the solution. You can settle your nervous system and improve your metabolism with something always available, regardless of your diet or environment, and it is your essential nature or true identity.

The physiological issues driving nervous system dysregulation are real. That's good news. Dysregulation means fluctuation. If something is making it worse, there must be something that can improve it. Every time you practice letting it be and relaxing the tension, you're allowing a feeling to move more freely, which is the beginning of bettering it. The more you remember to do it, the more you move in that direction. It might not feel like it immediately, but you're moving towards less suffering and more happiness, not because you are making anything come or go; you are simply uncovering what is already there. And you are improving how you feel and doing it by no longer doing what makes your system nervous.

Chapter 23 / What Me Worry About

A worry is a form of repetitive thinking that causes much suffering and unhappiness. But no matter what you worry about, the thing that causes suffering is not the specific worry itself but what you believe it means and how that makes you feel. The worry process happens quickly, often without you noticing it happening. Mostly it starts as a subtly unpleasant or uncomfortable feeling with a worried quality.

You worry about something by thinking about it. But, still, you feel worried and dislike how that feels, which adds tension, and then all of that makes you worry more about something by thinking about it. You think about how you don't like a feeling you think is there because of the thing that's bothering you. Then you think about how you want your worry to go away and how to make it go away. But that's just a diversion. You won't make a feeling go away by thinking about it.

On the contrary, that will make it more prominent and intense and can bring on an immense feeling like anxiety or panic. And then you'll think about it even more. The more you think about what you're worried about, the more nervous you are, so the more you worry. So you're strengthening a worry pathway.

When you feel worried, you always act a certain way; for example, calling a friend becomes part of your habitual reaction pattern. You think it's helping, but it's more distraction from feeling what you don't want to feel. Moreover, it makes it more likely you'll turn a feeling of worry into *The Feeling* again the next time it arises. If talking to a friend makes you feel better, you think it's because you solved the problem. But more often than not, the problem isn't the problem. The problem is resistance to a feeling, turning it into *The Feeling,* and hiding your essential self. You'll feel better when *The Feeling* eventually dissipates, but the next time a worry arises, you'll do the same again unless you learn to allow a feeling to be just a feeling.

A worried thought can arise first and bring on a feeling of worry, driving more thinking, emotion, and action. So the order is not the important thing. What's important is you can do this indefinitely if you never find out how it works. But when you find out, you can start undoing it.

Worry is very relevant to metabolism. Just look at what anxiety does to your stomach. Alternatively, you feel worried and realise it's just an upset stomach. Just an upset stomach can cause a lot of worries. It's only a feeling, but it's never too hard to find worrying material. Whatever pops into your thoughts will be what you're "worried about". Where were these thoughts when you weren't worried? Are these thoughts worrying, minus a feeling of worry?

> *Start worrying. Details to follow* (Text message from mum)

How many things can you worry about, and how many come true? If you worry about ten thousand things, and one of them comes true, is it right to worry? Or was all the worry worth it if you worry about one thing ten thousand times, and it eventually comes true?

Whether you worry about something or not depends on the personal story of you that you built. The details aren't the issue because the true you is not the story, and worry is an attempt to defend what is only relatively accurate and does not need defending. The story is at the heart of the subtle *craving* feeling, which brings up specific thoughts and emotions to support it. And they are thoughts and emotions that strengthen *The Feeling*. Wanting them gone is what makes them come back. So some people aren't worried about a thought that makes you panic. Not because of anything inherently worrying about it.

Worrying thoughts relate to a past or future event, but *The Feeling* takes place now. So that means you can fix a past or future event by dealing with *The Feeling*. For example, suppose anxiety arises, and you stop trying to control it. In that case, it will eventually burn itself out. Every time you do, it's as though you are undoing a past or future worry. It doesn't matter what the subject is. It's just a feeling you're fighting.

If a feeling of worry arises and you allow the energy to flow more freely, it will strengthen a habit of peace, calm and no worries resembling the true you. A worrying sensation is just energy flow inhibited, which hides your natural state. The natural flow of energy is blocked where this bad feeling resides. When thoughts get added to it, it doesn't matter if they're accurate. The story won't make it go away. Instead, it adds to the commotion.

> *'In shallow men the fish of little thoughts cause much commotion. In oceanic minds the whales of inspiration make hardly a ruffle.'* *This observation from the Hindu*

> *scriptures is not without discerning humor.* (Autobiography Of A Yogi Paramahansa Yogananda).

How you react to a feeling creates pathways or habits determining how much it makes you suffer. Depression, anxiety and panic go with metabolic dysfunction because the state of metabolism makes a particular kind of feeling arise. But the strength of the pathway to a specific type of reaction influences how far it will go. And it also affects the impact on metabolism. It's circular.

Illness is combined interferences with metabolic energy flow, bringing up a certain feeling. The more you resist it, the worse you feel, causing more interference. A feeling of worry is one such feeling, and the addition of all the layers makes you feel worse, and that can make you worry more, and then you get sick. And even if you recover fully, the experience will still leave a mark, strengthening a pathway. So then, the next time a feeling arises, it can trigger a chain reaction.

Worry habit gains momentum from the unwarranted reaction to a feeling of worry arising. It starts as just a little reaction, but then it grows. The reverse is also true. The choice to "unreact" can gradually reduce the momentum behind worry. Funny how the moment something you're worried about happens is the one moment you often worry the least. That is, until you start worrying about what's coming next.

Chapter 24 / Stress MetHabitolism

Metabolic stress is an unavoidable part of life, but habit powerfully influences the state of your metabolism. It's more like a MetHabitolism. If stress is your habit, then your metabolism will default to stress. And maybe you didn't know, but defaulting to stress is not the best way for metabolism to function, especially when exposed to stress. But this is still true even when stress exposure is low. Because there's stress, and then there's stress. There's the unavoidable initial stress and stress layered on top. So that's the stress it's good to be able to avoid.

But you can't just avoid it because you decide to avoid it. You have to know how to prevent it, and you have to be able to. Whether or not you can, has much to do with momentum. That's what a MetHabitolism is. It's a momentum mechanism in the process sense, not the machine sense. Everything metabolism is in process. Metabolism is a process. It is processing.

> *One who sees dependent origination sees the Dhamma; one who sees the Dhamma sees dependent origination.*
> (Mahāhatthipadopamasutta, Bhikkhu Bodhi, Majjhima Nikāya 28)

Momentum is what directs the process in a particular way. Whatever happens, influences what happens next. That's what the Buddha called "dependent origination". You might say small parts make up momentum. And together, they make something either more or less likely. How the next thing is, depends on how the last thing was. So even if you can't see it happening, it's happening. When momentum promotes stress, metabolism will deal with stress with more stress. Even if the stress isn't very stressful, it quickly becomes stressful. Then the pathway to a stress response becomes more robust.

To reverse the momentum, you need to be able to see what's happening. You can't rely on making stressful things not happen. Fixing diet and lifestyle helps up to a point. But every time a feeling arises, what happens next depends on the kind of MetHabitolism you have created.

It doesn't matter what feeling it is. Your MetHabitolism determines whether you're more likely to react to stress with stress or less likely.

The more you practice allowing stressful energy to flow unimpeded, the better you get at doing it, eventually, even with very stressful energy. And gradually, you change the direction of the momentum. Finally, you develop a habit of allowing stressful uncomfortable energy to flow through without interference. And then it no longer is stressful energy.

Stress is interference with the flow of energy. For example, when a feeling arises, and you identify with it and tense around it with dissatisfaction, you suppress the natural energy flow and increase stress. Stress is energy suppression because it interferes with thyroid energy metabolism.

"Expressing a feeling" can sound like a good idea, but it's dealing with stress by adding stress. Most of the time, you are expressing dissatisfaction with a feeling.

It's better to allow it to flow without interference. So when stress is high, you can take a step back, see what's beneath the layers, and then bring some "untensing" to the tension. Any time you do, and you feel some relief bubbling up, it's good to rest your attention there. This way, you become better acquainted with the healing energy always underneath stress. You can't control it, but you can allow it. It doesn't need controlling. It flows the way it flows; if you don't interfere, it will go the best way possible. Good or bad, now you aren't as attached.

Stress interferes with metabolism. It can interfere with brain energy homeostasis, glucose metabolism, and all metabolic processes. A relaxed metabolic state promotes a relaxed mind-body, and relaxing the mind-body promotes a relaxed metabolic state. So when a stressful feeling arises, and you allow it to flow, you are building a new habit that makes stress less stressful. It isn't new; you're uncovering your essential self. You're reversing momentum one stress at a time. You are using MetHabitolism in a way that benefits you. You create the momentum of allowing or letting things be as they are rather than what you want them to be. Then if a feeling arises, that's all it is, just a feeling. And you suffer less, and you're happier. Or happiness resurfaces.

Chapter 25 / "80% Perfect"

The best thing you can do now to feel better and improve your metabolism is to give up perfectionism. Right now. This minute. Please give it up completely. 100 per cent!

Yes, I'm joking, but not entirely. Perfectionism is a highly stressful condition, and it causes a great deal of suffering and unhappiness. There's a problem with perfectionism. It's a desire to create an ideal future free of dissatisfaction. But it's built on dissatisfaction with something happening now. Unfortunately, that's why it backfires.

As mentioned earlier, my yoga teacher often said, "80% Perfect". Most of the time, he was right because the primary thing yoga practice is for is not the reason most people practice. It helps you feel good, improves metabolic function, and settles the nervous system. It also helps with chronic digestive issues, depression, anxiety and other forms of inflammatory disease. And all this is especially true if you do it the right way. And there lies the paradox. Trying to do it correctly is the main thing preventing it from working correctly.

The fundamental purpose behind yoga is not to change how you feel. The real goal is to change *how you feel about how you feel*. It helps you to notice the layers that expand *The Feeling*. Its purpose is to bring you out of being lost in thinking and emotion so you can see the tension arising from dissatisfaction with a feeling and relax there. Perfectionism does the opposite.

Perfectionism is an attempt to make a feeling you are dissatisfied with go away or make a feeling you like to return and stay. That creates more tension and strengthens the pathway to perfectionism. If you achieve a perfectionist goal, the same perfectionism kicks in again. Lack of goal achievement isn't the problem, and goal achievement doesn't fix it.

The problem is that a feeling arises in the mind-body, and you want to control it. The problem is perfectionism. The story you tell yourself about creating the perfect future where the problem no longer exists is just a story. The story is part of the problem. You cannot make the ideal future because the attempt to create it makes the problem now, which drives the story about creating it. Every time you get there, the problem comes here with you. The projection into an imagined future creates tension in the present and does not feel good now, which is all there is and is already perfect.

In an imagined perfect future with excellent health, you can do the things you want to be able to do, and you can be happy. But, unfortunately, your current dissatisfaction with a feeling grows because of the attempt to make it go, and that's what makes you unhappy. It adds stress to a system struggling with stress. Stress is just an impersonal feeling. It is energy that sometimes doesn't feel great because of interference with its flow. It feels better without the layers, but it's easy to miss them getting added on. All that has to happen is for a feeling to arise. Then, before you know it, you tense up and escape into the fantasy world so quickly it feels like the story must be the way forward. But the story is only relatively accurate and hides the relief available here and now.

Once perfectionism becomes a habit, it won't rest until you attain it, which will never happen because striving for perfection hides perfection. You will, however, get perfect at detecting a feeling arising and reacting to it because that's the primary job of perfectionism. And there'll always be a feeling arising. So eventually, all you notice is what's wrong. No matter what you do, you can't make your metabolism perfect. You can't stop metabolic fluctuation, and you wouldn't want to. But you can easily create perfect dissatisfaction.

Chapter 26 / Symptoms Not Suffering

Most suffering results from reactions in the mind-body, from wanting less of a feeling you don't like or more of one you do like. Perhaps it sounds heartless to say it like that, but it's the opposite. The "heart" knows what to do. It's everything else that gets in the way. If you feel sadness and let it be sadness (easier said than done), it will go for as long as it goes until it dissipates. It won't always be fast, but it will be faster without the reaction to control it.

There's a big difference between a symptom and suffering or pain and suffering. A symptom is just a feeling. It can lead to suffering, but it depends on how you react. Two people can respond to the same pain very differently. One person can respond to the same pain differently depending on the circumstances. If you think pain is helping, for example, when you're working out, it won't bother you. However, if you believe pain is there because something is wrong, even if it isn't, it will feel very different. Some people barely react to any feeling that arises. Other people overreact to every sensation, ascribing detailed significance to each.

> *If God said, "Rumi, pay homage to everything that has helped you enter my arms," there would not be one experience of my life, not one thought, not one feeling, not any act, I would not bow to.*
> (Rumi)

My martial arts instructor used to say that reacting to

pain is a choice. And he seemed to practice what he preached under some extreme conditions. I'm not saying it's a good idea to ignore every feeling. The middle way is a better idea. But it's true; adding layers to pain is responsible for most suffering. So it's just a feeling, or it will be *The Feeling*. They're the only options.

Let's say you have a condition that causes pain and feel it daily. When the pain is there, the pain is there. That's the truth. How you react to it can be changed right now. And that's when the pain happens. If you don't like and want it gone, you're making it bigger and strengthening the pathway to more significant pain.

Stress and hypothyroidism are drivers of chronic pain. Tension, plus repetitive thinking and emotion, promote stress and thyroid dysfunction, which cause more tension and pain. It's science.

I'm not saying you should pretend to like pain. That's just more of the same controlling. But you can practice allowing it to be what it is without adding additional unnecessary parts. Thinking about why you don't want it to be there certainly won't make it go away.

Fear is another excellent example. A feeling of fear can arise for purely metabolic reasons or because of something you thought. Either way, what you do with it determines what happens next. A feeling of fear is the truth. It feels how it feels. It's the reaction to it that is a distortion. And that distortion is then the new truth, and how you react to that is another distortion. So you can get out of the way at any point, allowing it to flow more freely.

There will always be distortions. It's the nature of life. Metabolism is metabolising, for better or for worse. However, there's always a point where you can choose to be unattached. Even a system in a constant state of hyperreactivity to stress will benefit from allowing stress. That's true even after the best diet and lifestyle changes have largely failed. There will be a story of dissatisfaction and tension built into it. That's where you look. Happiness is hiding underneath.

That doesn't mean you'll make all symptoms disappear simply by stopping getting involved in the story. And it doesn't mean you don't act when you need to. Or eat what you think is best to eat. But the more you can disidentify with the personal story surrounding your pain, the less suffering and unhappiness it will bring, which can also help your metabolism heal.

There are many things you can do to improve how you feel. But a feeling is always just a feeling; pain is just a pain, and a symptom is just a symptom. Even suffering is just suffering. Once they are there, they are there, but what you do when they are there is everything. The more you resist them, the more they will fight you. And the further away you will get from relief.

Chapter 27 / Fear Of Fear

Most people think when they feel fear, it's because they're afraid of something they fear will happen. The truth is they're fearful of how they think it will feel if the thing they're scared of happens. And so there's fear. It is fear of a feeling. It can be sadness, anger, grief, depression, anxiety, disappointment or anything you feel. You feel fear about how something will feel in the future now. Now is the only time you can feel it. So think about that for a minute.

Fear arises, and fear is unpleasant. You don't like it, and you want it gone, and that causes tension, and then you think about things you fear. That creates more fear. You ruminate around what you fear because you think you can avoid feeling it by thinking about it, and then you feel the fear plus whatever gets added to it.

You end up feeling a combination of the original feeling of fear plus whatever gets added due to the tension and thinking. That's what *The Feeling* is; several parts get joined together. It's the full catastrophe feeling. Although it's still a feeling you can only feel now, it's painful and impacts metabolism more.

The rumination doesn't prevent anything you're afraid of from happening in the future. On the contrary, it makes you feel what you're scared of feeling in the future, over and over again. You feel it now, which is where you feel everything. I'm not the first to talk about this, but it's worth talking about because this tiny misunderstanding about what causes suffering and unhappiness causes so much suffering and unhappiness.

A feeling like fear can arise simply from eating something that causes a disturbance in the force. And then, before you know it, you're afraid and think you know why. You believe what you think you're scared of is what you fear. In one way, it is. But in another altogether different way, it isn't. Because a feeling of fear plus tension attaches itself to whatever pops into your head. That becomes what you're afraid of, and there doesn't have to be rhyme or reason. So the less you identify with what pops into your head, the less you'll be at the mercy of a feeling.

But we're taught to take the way we feel seriously, to honour how we feel. And we indeed should. But not in the way you might think. To honour how you feel, you have to allow how you feel to be how you feel. You do that more easily when you react to danger. But turning how you feel into your personal feeling is disrespectful. To respect how you feel, you don't interfere with how you feel. You don't turn it into something that it isn't out of fear of feeling it. If fear arises and you try to control it to avoid feeling it, you're just adding fear to fear. So what you have now is fear of fear, and it's multiple times scarier.

If you allow fear to flow unimpeded, it no longer feels like fear. *How you feel about how you feel* feels different from just a feeling. Raw fear feels more like any other natural feeling. Fear of fear is practically unrecognisable. A slightly negative and a somewhat positive sensation, minus the layers, are not that far apart. And it doesn't take much to shift from bad back to good. But projecting into the future (or the past) is the opposite of dealing with a feeling. You're trying to avoid it. That's what makes a feeling more challenging.

If a scary thought arises out of the blue that you want to get rid of, you can let it be there and treat it like it's just a thought passing through that has nothing to do with you. It's still energy, whether it's a thought or even an emotion. So if it's fear and you let it pass through, it will feel just like energy. It's fear of fear that induces the most fear. It's an idea about the past or the future that makes you feel fear now. This story of your fear is only relatively accurate, and no matter how big the fear gets or what solution you come up with, it happens now. And the way to solve it is to allow it. You can only feel a feeling now, so don't add to it; feel it now.

Chapter 28 / The Future Is Now

How you feel now is heavily influenced by how you think you will feel in the future, which then heavily influences how you feel in the future. And the influencing only ever takes place now. There's no worse position than trying to fix a future feeling because it doesn't exist yet. You cannot deal with a feeling that doesn't exist yet, now or ever. And yet a lot of energy is spent circling things that you're afraid will happen in the future and that will make you feel bad. And it makes you feel bad now.

There's an almost unlimited variety of experiences you can be afraid of experiencing. But, even so, people have their particular set of things that they circle, and the rest doesn't bother them much. So it doesn't make sense objectively. Why not be consistent and ruminate over everything according to likelihood or severity? For starters, you'd have little time left to do anything else. But some people come close to doing that. Even when they're doing something else, they're doing it. It doesn't make life very enjoyable.

The past and the future exist in your mind. So when something happens in your mind, it happens now. When you worry about the future, you feel the worry now, and so you experience it now. So even if the thing you're worried about never actually happens, it's already happened. Plus, you've also become more prone to feeling worried.

If you stop worrying about one thing, another will

replace it. All you need is a feeling of worry, and you immediately scan for something else to worry over. The more you practice worrying, the more you will bring it up. If you deal with something you were worried would happen so that you're no longer concerned about it, it will just get replaced with something else you find distressing.

The dealing isn't dealing. You just temporarily diverted from feeling what you don't want to feel, and there's no shortage of things you haven't dealt with yet. I'm not saying you can't fix a problem. There's nothing wrong with doing that. But ultimately, what you are worried about lies under every story, and starts to disappear when you face and release it. It's *craving*, the fictional story of you and your vulnerability. Repetitive thinking creates more problems than it solves because the problem is not the real problem. The real problem is what you feel and what you think it means. And you can start to deal with that by feeling that. It's *The Feeling* that is the problem, not just a feeling. *The Feeling* prevents you from feeling a feeling.

You can do something to fix something if and when it can get fixed. For example, if you want to improve how you hit a tennis ball, you must wait for it to come over the net to practice hitting it. You can even do some imagining as a form of practice. But there's a difference between practising and worrying about whether you'll hit the ball well, how you'll feel if you fail, what that will do to your tennis career, and so on. And if you're worried you won't be able to stop all this circular worrying, don't worry; you don't have to. You don't even want to try. That's what makes it happen more. It's just another feeling happening now that you're trying to control. It's the same habit. What you need to deal with to feel better in the future is how you feel now. If you worry now, you also worry when you reach your new future. That's how it works.

> *Let not a person revive the past,*
> *Or on the future build his hopes,*
> *For the past has been left behind,*
> *And the future has not been reached.*
> *Instead with insight (wisdom) let him see*
> *Each presently arisen state; Let him know*
> *that and be sure of it, Invincibly,*
> *unshakably.*
> *Today the effort must be made;*
> *Tomorrow Death may come, who knows?*
> *No bargain with Mortality can keep him*
> *and his hordes away, But one who dwells*
> *thus ardently,*
> *Relentlessly, by day, by night--*
> *It is he, the 'Peaceful Sage' has said.*
> *Who has had a single excellent night* (MN 131 Bhaddekaratta Sutta, Bhikkhu Bodhi).

Thankfully, to deal with how you feel now, you don't have to deal with anything. It's more like you have to "un-deal" with it. Dealing with it is what creates tension in the first place. It's because you want to control it to avoid feeling it. It's a diversion tactic. But when you divert from it, you miss out on seeing what's underneath, peace.

So relax the tension that comes with a feeling. Release it, let it flow, and relax right there. That's how you fix the future, by fixing how you feel now. Because now is when the future happens. There will always be problems to solve, and bad things happen, so there'll also always be a new problem to replace a problem. So the potential for suffering and unhappiness is practically unlimited. Fortunately, there is only one moment where you need to deal with it. And all you need to do is allow it.

It's like magic. And so it also works for fixing the past. You can't change what happened; you can change how you feel about it now. You allow how you feel now to be how you feel. If you fully feel how you feel now, it's just a feeling about the past, and you've changed the past. Now.

Chapter 29 / Habitual Pathways

No metabolic issue is continuous, but the appearance of metabolic continuity is created one interaction at a time. That's how to manufacture and maintain a chronic problem. One stress at a time. Stress causes interference with metabolism, and interference with metabolism causes stress, which drives more interference with metabolism. It's just basic maths, and there's a new opportunity to change the interaction every moment.

Stress pathways created over time build up a lot of momentum, so much so that even when metabolism improves, stress can remain the baseline for a long time. But regardless, every moment, you have an opportunity to either react to stress with more stress or with more allowing. Not perfect allowing at first, but even little bits of allowing can eventually build momentum in the direction of allowing.

Allowing is the opposite of stress. Or, at the very least, it's how you meet stress to avoid turning (unavoidable) stress into excessive stress or distress. The more you strive to improve metabolic health, the more you intensify the things that make you want to strive to improve metabolic health in the first place. Because interference with metabolism drives metabolic issues, and interference with metabolism does not just come down to the state of your metabolism.

The state of your metabolism is more than just the state of your metabolism. It's not separate from everything else around you. Diet, environment, lifestyle factors, and your emotional or psychological condition come to mind. So the state of your metabolism influences your psychology, and the state of your metabolism is affected by your psychology.

Which came first, the chicken or the egg? They both did. But it doesn't matter so much. Your ability to choose how you react to a feeling provides an ongoing opportunity to influence your psychology and metabolism. Every time you become aware of this opportunity, you get a chance to add stress or to de-stress. And every time you become aware of this opportunity, you recognise that you are more than your mind-body and increase the likelihood that you will become aware of this opportunity again next time.

The problem is when you don't like the way you feel. It's natural to strive to feel better. You hear how to make yourself feel better and automatically go at it with gusto. And that's the trap. You want it to work. And built into the wanting it to work is the not wanting it not to work. So it's got the tension that helped get you here in the first place, inside it. It's a subtle trap that can easily trap you even after you know about it. Because there's knowing, and then there's knowing. Intellectual knowing is easy, but more is needed. The knowing that works best comes from experience. When you step back, you experience your true nature, and it's more than the story of your likes and dislikes and what they represent. But the story can still be true relatively.

You need to know how to fix what's wrong with you while also knowing that fixing is the thing that is wrong with you. There's no riddle. You have to get your head around that. It's like the Magic Eye again. It's right there in front of you, but you're getting in your way. You're always fixing without realising it, and that's what you need to fix. Fixing becomes the normal state. It's not one long continuous fixing, but lots of tiny fixings. You won't catch them all, but it doesn't matter. Starting is what matters—and continuing.

> *Most of our efforts, most of our intentions and our search are for saying `I am different from that which I feel, and how am I to resolve that?'. This is really an important issue not to be easily brushed aside and cunningly replied. You have to look at it though your whole being revolts; because we have been brought up to think that you can operate on it. You are not at all a different entity from your thought or from your desire or your ambition, from the ladder you are climbing, spiritually or sociologically. To understand this problem there must be communion with the whole, and you cannot commune with the whole if you are looking at it partially as you and the object.* (Jiddu Krishnamurti, 1952)

Every arising feeling can be a trigger to set off stress. Or it can be a trigger to remember to allow. It's just a feeling that doesn't feel how you want it to, and fighting it causes it to grow. It helps to treat a feeling the way you'd treat an angry or upset child. For example, suppose you meet them with upset or anger. That might temporarily suppress their reaction, but that's not the way to get a healthy resolution. And for sure don't tell them their problems aren't as big as they think. When you meet a feeling with an allowing mindset, you're meeting it but getting out of its way simultaneously. And you are taking it less seriously. You're letting it do its thing, like a healthy metabolism meeting stress. That doesn't block the energy; it allows it to flow. And it leads to metabolic equilibrium.

A healthy metabolism does not get rid of stress. Instead, it recognises it, and it allows it so that it doesn't cause more stress than necessary. Then stress still happens when there is stress. It just doesn't turn into a habit.

Chapter 30 / Smiling Lowers Serotonin

According to the official narrative, serotonin is the happiness chemical. Still, the truth is that couldn't be further from the truth. Smiling lowers serotonin, as well as other substances that also do not promote happiness.

The defensive chemicals (including serotonin) rise under stress conditions and smiling lowers stress substance release. When you reduce stress, you smile more. Like all things mind-body or metabolism, it works both ways.

Indeed, it doesn't feel natural to smile when you don't feel like smiling, just like it doesn't feel natural to relax when you aren't, but that doesn't mean it isn't a good idea. It's a type of reverse engineering for happiness. When you feel happy, you smile, and so it stands to reason that when you smile, you'll feel happy. It's simple but not always easy. For example, the last thing you want to do when you're unhappy is force yourself to smile. And as you know, using force is not the best way to improve how you feel.

Luckily there's no need for any force. Just start lifting the sides of your mouth a bit when you remember. You don't have to start with times when you're especially miserable, although there'd be no harm in that. Just lifting the sides of your mouth pretty immediately encourages a smiling mind-body, and a smiling mind-body is an allowing mind-body. When you smile (a smile on the outside and the inside), you help energy flow freely or with less interference. That's why it feels good even when things don't feel so good. But smiling when you're not happy won't feel natural at first. It won't immediately fix all your issues or free up all the energy blockages. It will, however, immediately reduce resistance to a feeling you're resisting.

> *Smiling and/or laughing, whether you feel like it or not, can have an immediate effect on your metabolism. You might not notice it straight away, but after a while you will start to see the truth in this statement.* (Me)

When there's less resistance to a resisted feeling, there's increased allowing of the flow of energy. Interference with energy flow causes stress to become a problem. Stress itself isn't the problem per se. Instead, how you meet stress determines its impact. If stress is unmet or resisted, then that will promote more interference with energy flow.

Serotonin interferes with energy flow. When the demands of stress are unable to be met, serotonin rises to limit metabolic damage by temporarily reducing energy demands. Serotonin suppresses metabolism so that fewer functions that require energy are functioning. It is protective in the short term, but it isn't optimal. If high stress is ongoing, serotonin can cause stress issues, including depression and anxiety.

Serotonin closes you down, and smiling opens you up. Serotonin promotes interference with energy. Smiling promotes allowing. If thyroid metabolism is optimal, you meet stress with allowing. The result is an opening up to experience. When you're closed off to experience, you suffer more and are less happy. It's because you respond to a feeling with *craving* and then the other layers. Metabolically, an experience is energy demand. A closed metabolism means stress substances like serotonin rise in response to demand. As a result, the use of sugar is interfered with, reducing nutritional requirements.

Serotonin is the "hibernation chemical". Hibernation is metabolic suppression in defence against stress or scarcity. It is torpor, not restful sleep, which requires more energy. Serotonin rises for survival, but surviving is not the same as surviving optimally. Smiling opens you up to experience and supports energy flow. Smiling supports thyroid metabolism. Thyroid and smiling both promote the ability to relax. Relaxation is a high-energy state, whereas low-energy availability promotes tension, excitation, and stress. Everything makes more sense this way. Optimal thyroid, relaxation and happiness go together; they are the same.

Serotonin is the avoidance chemical. It encourages the avoidance of stress because a demand feels too high to handle. However, a higher-functioning system can handle the same stress without suppression or avoidance. Smiling is the opposite of avoidance. The more you smile, the more stress you can handle. Avoidance promotes interference with energy flow, and that fosters depression and anxiety and other forms of suffering.

Smiling signals the free movement of energy; when it moves freely, it feels good, making you smile more. There's no mystery here. You cannot avoid the arising of a feeling, but you can take things less personally.

Serotonin makes things personal. Smiling is the opposite of taking things personally. The more you smile, the less everything is about you and your story of "things you like and things you dislike". Smiling uncovers your true nature.

> *So you put a little smile on your lips. You smile in your mind of course, you smile with your eyes even when you have your eyes closed. That lets go of a lot of tension. And you smile in your heart. So the more you smile the more uplifted your mind becomes, the more uplifted your mind becomes, the more you start to experience joy arising.* (Venerable Bhante Vimalaramsi)

As a bonus, things that happen metabolically, making you smile more, happen more when you smile more. But, again, this is because smiling helps allow a feeling to be just a feeling.

Chapter 31 / Serious Anxiety And Depression

Anxiety and depression can be serious issues. One of the main reasons for this is that they thrive on taking things seriously. That probably sounds harsh and uncaring, but take a moment to contemplate it. Of course, anxiety and depression have a variety of forces involved in their progression. Still, in every case, for anxiety and depression to become serious issues, there must be a certain amount of taking things seriously.

If you subtract all the reasons you're anxious or depressed, all that's left is how you feel. Why a feeling arises varies from one situation to another and one person to another. But every feeling starts as just a feeling. *The Feeling* is the Frankenstein version of a feeling. It's just a feeling, but it gets turned into a monster, and the monster wreaks havoc. The *craving* reaction to its arising makes a feeling morph into a monster. *Craving* is taking things seriously. You don't like it, and it shouldn't be happening; to you.

There's nothing inherently wrong with fear or sadness, for example. But you don't like it, and you have a lot of reasons why you want it gone. And they're serious reasons. There's nothing wrong with that, as long as you know that's what makes just a feeling grow into anxiety or depression. You build anxiety and depression by trying not to allow what's happening to happen. Of course, you don't want it to happen, but unfortunately, that makes it grow.

Metabolic issues, like excess exposure to serotonin, drive depression and anxiety. And diet and lifestyle changes that improve thyroid metabolism are powerfully protective. The right changes make a person feel much better and often reduce the size and length of episodes of depression and anxiety. Even so, depression and anxiety can be like a creature that raises its head when the opportunity presents itself. That has much to do with how a person habitually reacts to a feeling. There can be powerful momentum behind these reactions, which is strengthened by how personally you take it. Or, in other words, how serious you believe it is.

So the antidote is to see the fiction added to it, which can be difficult to do when everything feels serious. Your experiences are still your experiences, and your pain is still real. None of this is about denial. But ultimately, you are not what you experience, and if you decide you have suffered enough, this is the way forward. Ironically this way leads to proper validation of suffering. It means not fighting with suffering and allowing it to be what it is. Then it isn't suffering anymore. It's just a feeling that you experience. It's trying to control suffering that causes the most suffering. So taking it too seriously fuels more thoughts about suffering, which fuels the expansion of *The Feeling*.

> *Everything that arises, every thought, every feeling that arises, is impersonal. Nobody is going to say, "Well, I haven't been depressed for a long time. I haven't been sad for a long time. I haven't been highly emotional for a long time. I guess I might as well have some now." Nobody says that! It happens because the*

> *conditions are right for these kinds of things to arise. What you do with them right now dictates what happens in the future* (Venerable Bhante Vimalaramsi).

No matter how you feel, the addition of *how you feel about how you feel* and the other layers make how you feel far more unpleasant. And there's practically no limit to how unpleasant you can make it feel. But how much of this belongs to your true essence? How you feel is not static; how you interpret it is accurate roughly the same way a broken clock is correct, only occasionally. But if you take it all seriously, it feels like it must always be right.

This whole process is circular and stressful. It promotes stress substances like serotonin, and everything seems serious when stress and serotonin are high. It makes you less open to experience, so you trap yourself in a particular version. That's the version that is the story of you. The more you think about your story, the more likely you will get anxious and depressed. Stepping back from thoughts and feelings allows them to move through more freely. You don't have to like them. You don't have to do anything apart from letting them be. If you still don't like them, you can let that be too. The less you get involved, the less personal it is; it creates a non-vicious circle.

The more you try to control how you feel, the more you grow a sense of self. Lowering stress and promoting thyroid metabolism lowers serotonin and promotes opening up to the world. It helps you take everything less seriously and removes some of the separations between yourself and others. And that helps a lot with depression and anxiety. Optimal thyroid is allowing and impersonal; serotonin makes things personal; it resists stress. And resistance to stress equals suffering. But please don't take my word for it. The beauty of this is it's easily testable. But remember, don't take the testing too seriously, either. Or the results. If you do, you might end up summoning Dr Frankensteins' monster again, and nobody needs that.

Chapter 32 / Reverse Superstition

Almost every superstition you have will get proven right, eventually. And when it does, you'll forget about the other 999,999 times it got proven wrong. That's why it can be so hard to let go of superstition. It's self-reinforcing. You ignore the times the thing you fear doesn't come to pass and remember the times it does. It's a powerful form of cognitive bias. Of course, cognition can't help but be biased, but reducing superstition makes you happier, so it's worth a look.

Superstition works a lot like Obsessive-compulsive disorder (OCD). It's essentially the same process. The process works like this. You think you must do something a certain way or something terrible will happen. If you do the thing and nothing bad happens, that reinforces the belief that doing the thing is why nothing bad happened. And if something terrible happens, you must not have done the thing the right way. Otherwise, it wouldn't have happened.

But what about times when you didn't do the thing, and nothing bad happened? You ignore them because they don't count! That's cognitive bias at work. It can be repeating a phrase, spinning around in a circle, checking you turned off the stove fifty times before you leave, or tapping the door seven times after you shut it. It's the same process for all of them. Logically speaking, it doesn't add up, but it just takes being right that one time to reinforce the habit powerfully.

It's really about control. You fear something will

happen, and you think if you do the thing, you'll prevent what you fear from happening. You think it works because it makes you feel better when a feeling you don't like arises. You're just reacting to a feeling that's happening now, that you connect to thoughts about the future, and your reaction works to make you feel better, temporarily. And when it doesn't make you feel better, the solution is to add more things to the things you do: an extra circle, a few more taps, or an additional phrase. The possibilities are endless.

It doesn't fix the problem because it doesn't deal with the cause. And every time you deal with what you think is the cause, another feeling is waiting to pop up. That's all the inspiration you need for the whole thing to start again.

So the issue is it's all just a diversion from dealing with the issue. And the issue is the same issue it always is. A feeling arises, and you tense up around it, take it personally and try to control it. The things you do to push a feeling away reinforce the habit of pushing it away. But 99.99% of the things you think you will control don't happen. And the things that do happen happen regardless of the rituals. So it's a big waste of time and energy, and it causes suffering and unhappiness rather than preventing it.

There is a solution. I call it "Reverse Superstition". You do the opposite of what you've been doing and untangle the mess bit by bit. When you feel the urge to do the thing, you notice the dissatisfaction and allow it to be there. Then, you "untense" the tension, stop controlling how you feel and let the energy pass through. "Untensing" tension is more like undoing than doing.

You release your hold on it. If you were squeezing a ball and you suddenly noticed you're squeezing it and that it's causing tension, you wouldn't need instructions. You'd stop squeezing. You'd let go and let it rest in your hand. Then you'd feel relief. That's what it feels like to let go.

> *Don't think. Feel. It's like a finger pointing at the moon. Do not concentrate on the finger, or you will miss all of the heavenly glory* (Bruce Lee, Enter The Dragon)

Don't squeeze. Let go. Don't concentrate on the tension; you'll miss all the heavenly relief. Don't focus too hard on the relief, but you can always bask in it. It's your true nature. It's an antidote to stress. It's a sign you're allowing energy metabolism to flow. And it's an antidote to superstition and repetitive thinking. Repetitive thinking is just another form of superstition or OCD. You fear something will happen in the future, and you think if you think about it, you'll prevent the thing you fear from happening. But no matter how many different ways you think about it, you're missing what's causing it, which is just a feeling happening now, with a story added. All you want is to feel better now. It has nothing to do with the future or the past.

When letting go of control becomes your new habit, you see how you constantly react to a feeling. There isn't anything you need to control because nothing has happened. When something does happen, it has already happened. It's only superstition that keeps the superstition going. It's the OCD that keeps the OCD going. Avoidance of a feeling prevents it from resolving. That's all it prevents.

Superstition is the opposite of allowing. It's taking a feeling personally and then taking the story you build on that seriously. Then you have no choice but to act. But you are not the story. "Reverse Superstition" creates the habit of allowing a feeling to be just a feeling. Then you can uncover your true self and act when acting is appropriate.

Chapter 33 / Pain Is Impermanent

The hardest thing about believing pain is impermanent is believing it when you're in pain. And unfortunately, that's when you need to believe it most. When I say pain, I mean any painful feeling. It can be a feeling of anxiety or sadness or nausea, or muscular pain. When pain arises, it is hard not to focus on it; when you focus on it, it's hard not to think about it. Because you think you can make the pain disappear by thinking about it. But pain doesn't work that way.

Thinking about it is an attempt to escape feeling it, but you always get recaptured and punished. The punishment is that the pain gets worse and becomes more permanent. What's happening is pain is being strengthened one layer at a time, and that makes it more likely to continue from one moment to the next. I'm not suggesting you ignore pain or that you can prevent pain from happening or make it go away, but things are constantly in flux. So that means pain must either get better or worse or stay roughly the same. So pain is never a fixed thing.

Metabolism isn't a fixed thing, either. But, likewise, neither is suffering, unhappiness, or any feeling that arises. So it means *how you feel about how you feel* impacts the direction of the flux, the pathway, the momentum, and other ways of describing it. They're just descriptions, but help point your attention in the right direction. Your attention always points somewhere. Just because there's pain doesn't mean you must put all your attention there and make it a big deal. When you do, it adds stress on top of stress, making it more stressful.

> *The more we escape, the greater and more complex the problems become. When we look at the problem, our whole structure is a series of escapes. You explain away sorrow; to you then, explanation has more significance than the depth, the meaning, the vitality of sorrow. After all, the explanations are merely words, however subtle, however justified; and we are satisfied with words. This is another escape.* (Jiddu Krishnamurti, 1952)

Not making a big deal out of pain does not mean denying the existence of pain. On the contrary, focusing all your attention on pain and denying the fact of pain are both attempts to escape feeling pain, and you can't run forever. And it's escaping that makes something impermanent into something more permanent. The alternative is allowing. Or else it's called releasing or letting go or softening or relaxing. It has lots of names. They all mean the same. You see a pain has arisen, and instead of reacting with dissatisfaction, tension, and all the other layers, you "unreact". You let go of your grip on it, improving energy flow. You know it's there but don't hone in on it. You don't become it because you know you are more than it.

Blocked or inhibited energy creates the illusion of permanence because meeting stress with more stress makes it stronger and last longer than it otherwise would. It can stop it from being able to resolve. That's how metabolism works, and that's why it's called metabolism because it's metabolising. So it's either improving or staying roughly the same or worsening. And even if it's deteriorating, it can happen quickly or slowly. The word metabolism is related to the Greek "to change". Metabolism is constantly changing. The last change impacts every change. So it's dependently arising, just like the Buddha said.

You think of it as "your pain", but the personalisation of pain is what can make an impermanent pain more permanent. The thing is, it's a different pain from one moment to the next. But the more you focus on it and identify with it as your pain that is part of what's wrong with you, the more painful it is, and the longer it's likely to stick around. Building a story around pain creates more stress and tension, hiding what is always available; relaxation, happiness or loving-kindness. Please don't take my word for it. You can find out for yourself.

The solution isn't to deny pain. It's to allow pain to be what it is, just a feeling. When pain is just a pain that's there, and it's allowed to be that, it expresses itself more accurately and dissipates more quickly. And if it doesn't, it's still just pain. It's something happening in the mind-body but does not define you. The more you ruminate and the more meaning you give to it, the more momentum it will have behind it. It's like artificial permanence. It's the opposite of being kind to yourself. Resisting or fighting pain causes you pain.

You still can't control pain, but if you understand the laws of metabolism, you can get out of the way and stop adding problems on top of something already there. Nevertheless, a painful feeling has arisen, and that's a fact. Figuring out why it has arisen is helpful up to a point. Sometimes treatment is necessary. Still, once figuring out becomes personalising, controlling, contracting, disliking, and bargaining, it uses much more energy. You make the best decisions minus the clutter. Feeling, thinking, and acting are alright, but the more attached you are, the bigger and more permanent a feeling becomes.

You prevent healing with control. The less interference, the more resilience because resilience means being comfortable with what is uncomfortable. And more resilience means less suffering and more happiness. A good feeling comes out of uninhibited energy flow. So it's good to put some attention there lightly. That's the closest thing to control without controlling because you become more aware of your energetic self and allow it to flow. It can feel like permanence, but it's pure impermanence, the only thing that isn't impermanent. And it is your essential nature.

Chapter 34 / Catch a Bad Mood

A bad mood is a condition that passes from one person to the next, but the truth is that you don't need to be around other people to get into one. You can do it well enough on your own. Your mood is impacted by how you feel, but it's even more powerfully affected by *how you feel about how you feel*. Add thinking, emotion, and action into the mix, and you have an explosive mood-worsening cocktail.

The reverse is also true. Your mood influences how you feel and *how you feel about how you feel*, and it affects your thoughts, emotions and actions. Like most things mind-body, it's circular. And like most things in the mind-body, it's driven by momentum or habit. So it can be challenging to change from being someone who defaults to unhappy into someone who defaults to happy.

Mood can drive feelings and thoughts, and they can then drive mood, and round and round it goes. So it's normal, and it's why *The Feeling* is self-feeding. But the more you practice noticing what creates *The Feeling*, the more you will see what's fueling its momentum. Then you can start letting go of your hold on it all and stop adding to the bad mood habit.

But, of course, you will still need to cultivate a new habit, the good mood habit. Undoing existing momentum is not enough because attention is always going somewhere. So attention gets pulled to what's left of the old habit when the opportunity arises. That can prevent a new one from being formed. Don't worry, though. You don't have to perform magic and make a good feeling appear out of thin air. The good mood energy is always there; it's your fundamental nature. But it's inhibited because you're squeezing. So you have to release your hold a bit, and the better the energy will flow. That is an opportunity to cultivate a more "wholesome", more relaxed momentum.

When a good feeling arises, you can loosely place your attention in that general direction and enjoy it while it lasts. Don't try to control or make it stay. Just bask in it. It's healing energy, so the more time you spend with it, the more it will stick around, and the easier it will be for it to arise again. It never went anywhere; healing thyroid energy is what you are, in essence, but it gets suppressed. The more familiar it becomes, the more you meet stress with thyroid energy, so it doesn't become "distress". A good mood comes out of uninhibited energy flow. Conversely, inhibiting energy flow worsens mood.

Take other people, for example. They can be the source of a worsening mood. It's like their mood is contagious. But like all things contagion, how their attitude impacts your mood has as much to do with you as with them. When you come into contact with another person, you can feel the energy of how they feel passing to you, and it feels like something you feel directly. It truly is contagious in that sense. You can feel it. But remember, how you feel is just a feeling, so the issue is what happens afterwards.

What does it do to *how you feel about how you feel*, what you think, your emotions, and what you say and do? Then what do you think all that will do? I'll tell you what it doesn't do. If a person is stressed and you get stressed because they're stressed, that won't make them less stressed. Instead, it will just increase the stress for both of you. You become one combined mind-body, creating a more powerful escalation of *The Feeling*. That's just two people. Imagine a big group.

People also think they can eliminate a bad mood by communicating it to another person. They believe sharing the story makes *The Feeling* go away. Maybe it feels like that. You can pass a feeling to others, which may make you feel better temporarily. Still, it can be another version of symptom suppression. It feels like it's working, but if you don't recognise the actual cause, the *craving*, you can increase the problem over time.

> *Some planets rolled in those openings on the side of my head. I haven't heard anything for years.*
> *Whenever I see a mouth moving in front of me I just assume someone is saying something brilliant and then go on about my day feeling very secure* (Tukaram)

Another common way is to burn off a bad mood by replacing it with a feeling you find more manageable, like replacing sadness with anger, for example. Maybe someone you care about is upset, and you don't like how that feels, so you react with anger. Unfortunately, this way is prevalent, but it also backfires. It's far from being a pro-metabolic mindset. Even though the mood is contagious, how you react changes everything for you and others. How you treat others might as well be how you treat yourself; ultimately, it is. And it adds fuel to the momentum behind stress. And more stress makes you more susceptible to contagion.

A bad mood is similar to a metabolic issue. It's just a feeling that arises. Once it appears, you make it worse if you use force to try and control it. Like any bad feeling, a bad mood thrives on resistance. What you have to do is let it flow. The same applies to the mood of another person. You can't make it go away, and you can't take it from them. But you can allow it to flow through you by not resisting it, which will likely help it flow through them too.

Chapter 35 / Which Meditation?

The Buddha taught a different kind of meditation. He mastered the practices of the day, and he found them to be less than satisfying. It wasn't until discovering how to allow a feeling that he knew he was finally on the right path. He also knew what the right way wasn't. For example, he discovered that using meditation to stop thoughts, empty your mind, or make a bad feeling go away, can feel great. But it does so with suppression.

And it's easy to get fooled by suppression results because it can quickly make painful symptoms disappear. Once you have an experience like that, it's hard to let go of it, even long after it stops working. Because the pain went away, you think the pain was the thing causing all the suffering. When it went away, the suffering went away with it. That's the dream, which is what it is—a dream. Or maybe fantasy is more accurate.

When the pain comes back, and it will, the suffering will come back with it. Maybe even more potent because now it comes with added stress. You thought you were better. It's disappointing and stressful. So the obvious thing to do now is to do what worked before but do it even better this time. Try harder, suppress more. You know it works. You have to get it to work more. The reality is that it's only a temporary fix. And the fixing causes the situation to get worse.

The Buddha discovered that's because there is *craving* built into the fixing. You don't like how you feel and want to make a bad feeling disappear. So the Buddha realised that *craving* was the real cause of suffering and unhappiness. But to understand that, you must realise that you can't make the pain disappear. When it's there, it's there, and there will always be pain; suffering comes from identifying with and then fighting with that reality.

None of this has anything to do with getting rid of desire or pleasure or anything for that matter. You can have all of those things, either with or without *craving*. Trying to get rid of them is *craving*. It's about the story attached to it. You want it because you think you'll find happiness there, but it's not there. The same applies to metabolic health. You can't make a metabolism free of fluctuation because metabolism is fluctuation. You may as well bang your head against a brick wall. It's OK to do the things that improve metabolic health, but essentially, what you are is metabolism. When you think you can use what you are to control what you are, you are heading in the direction of stress. When stress gets too high, you suffer more.

So this book is not a guidebook for attaining perfect metabolic health unless, by perfect metabolic health, you mean perfect allowing metabolism to be what it is— a metabolism. And ultimately, metabolism always is perfect; it only gets resisted.

This book is not a meditation instruction manual. I'm not a meditation expert or an expert on Buddhism or spirituality. Nor is it a positive thinking self-help book. These books often fail because most methods promoted for fixing health and well-being rely on suppression to get results. Suppression works well when everything goes according to plan, but it all starts to fall apart as soon as things get chaotic.

What's written was influenced by the teachings of the Buddha (and others) and the guidance of Venerable Bhante Vimalaramsi. Bhante developed Tranquil Wisdom Insight Meditation (TWIM) based on his understanding of the Buddha's teachings (taken from the Buddhist suttas) and his direct experience. I have practised TWIM for a few years and highly recommend it to reduce suffering and increase happiness and metabolic function. I recommend it regardless of metabolism.

Any kind of meditation practice can be highly beneficial. Still, if it works as a form of suppression, the things you suppress will return when you are not meditating. And then you'll think, "What happened?". I know what happened. You stopped a feeling, taking your suffering away and making you happy. Then a feeling came back. You don't need more suppression because that's what got you here in the first place. Instead, it would help if you had a new habit built on a new way of relating to whatever arises.

> *I was meditating with my cat the other day and all of a sudden she shouted, "What happened?" I knew exactly what she meant, but encouraged her to say more—feeling that if she got it all out on the table she would sleep better that night. So I responded, "Tell me more, dear," and she soulfully meowed, "Well, I was mingled with the sky. I was comets whizzing here and there. I was suns in heat, hell—I was galaxies. But now look— I am landlocked in fur." To this I said, "I know exactly what you mean." What to*

say about conversation between mystics?
(Tukaram)

Meditation practice helps, but it's a meditation practice for a reason. You're practising for the main event. It's like you want to learn high diving. But you're afraid whenever you get to the top and look over the edge. So you stand there frozen. And you suffer. Instinctively you know there's water at the bottom and that all you have to do is jump, and you will get the relief you are after, but you're afraid of what will happen. Meditation is practising on a low board with floaties on. It's lots of little jumps; the big jumps will eventually be easy.

Whether or not you have fur, you're landlocked in the mind-body, and that's how it is. You can get the best out of that by becoming comfortable with the fluctuations that always come with it. The more comfortable you are, the less extreme the fluctuations, and you're more likely to find what you want. That is less suffering and more happiness. It is the middle way and helps you see that the answer is always there because you are it.

Printed in Great Britain
by Amazon